Holistic
Living

A guide to self-care

Dr Patrick Pietroni

J. M. Dent & Sons Ltd
London Melbourne

First published 1986
© Patrick Pietroni 1986

This book is set in 9½/11pt Palatino Roman by
Input Typesetting Ltd

Printed in Great Britain by The Guernsey Press Co. Ltd,
Guernsey, C.I. for
J. M. Dent & Sons Ltd
Aldine House, 33 Welbeck Street, London W1M 8LX

British Library Cataloguing in Publication Data

Pietroni, Patrick
  Holistic living: a guide to self-care.—
  (Healthright)
  1. Holistic medicine
  I. Title II. Series
  613   R733

  ISBN 0–460–02414–0

Contents

Preface

It has been over three years since Prince Charles addressed the British Medical Association's annual conference and suggested that 'Human nature is such that we are frequently prevented from seeing that what is taken for today's unorthodoxy is probably to be tomorrow's convention'. He went on to add that

> The whole imposing edifice of modern medicine, for all its breathtaking successes, is like the celebrated Tower of Pisa, slightly off-balance.

It could be said that the human condition is one in which we are all constantly striving to remain on-balance. The sudden surge of interest in alternative/complementary medicine, self-help approaches to health, diet-conscious shopping, jogging clubs etc. is all an attempt to look for ways of restoring our balance.

The British Holistic Medical Association was set up in 1983 as an organisation for doctors and medical students wishing to expand their understanding of Holistic Medicine. Since then it has grown to include both complementary practitioners as well as the 'public'. The words 'complementary/alternative' and 'holistic' are often misunderstood and one of the principal reasons for writing this book was to help explain what holism is about. It certainly is not against orthodox medicine nor is it a wholesale application of alternative therapies. The need to balance 'specialism' with an understanding of how we are all part of one 'whole' is a pressing need in medicine. This need is finding voice in many other areas of our life. The most recent disaster at Chernobyl is a dramatic illustration of how our global village has become a stark reality. We live in a participatory world and we can no longer continue to live as if we were isolated, independent individuals, let alone isolated independent countries. The search for wholeness has to be conducted both within ourselves and with our fellow human beings. It is a search that will no doubt continue for as long as man remains divided and at war with himself.

My own search continues and the book I would write in ten years' time would hopefully be different from this first attempt to outline my own current understanding. This book is a bringing together of the many guides and teachers who have helped me on my way. It owes much to my family and friends who have tolerated my many 'departures' and 'side-tracks' I have taken in my haste to find 'the answer'. It is also a testimony to the patience, guidance and friendship of my wife, without whom it would not have been written.

An audio-cassette recording of several exercises described in this book is available from the British Holistic Medical Association, 179 Gloucester Place, London NW1 6DX

Acknowledgments

The author and publishers would like to thank the following for permission to quote material:

Sphere Books Ltd: a table from Peter Lambley, *Insomnia*.
The National Heart Foundation of Australia: an appendix from *Guide to Exercise*.
Macdonald and Co. (Publishers) Ltd: tests from *BUPA Manual of Fitness and Well-being*.
Crown Publishers, Inc.: *Visual Encyclopaedia*.

1

WHAT IS HOLISM?

'Holism is about being holy,' 'It's about yoga, jogging and yogurt', 'It's about "alternative medicine"'. These are some of the common statements that have been made about this new word that has crept into our language in the last few years. Often when it is necessary to define a new concept or approach, it can be helpful to describe what it is not and although some of those statements mentioned above are near to the definition of holism, they are also very far from a true description.

Holism is essentially about an approach each of us can use to help us understand ourselves and our place in the world in which we live. From this deeper understanding we can begin to make more informed choices about our health and the way we conduct our lives. The 'spectacles' we put on to view ourselves and the world determine the sort of picture we see. If we put on a 'blue pair' of spectacles, all we see will look blue. Similarly, if we put on a 'yellow pair' the world will look yellow. If we put on a holistic pair of spectacles then some of the difficulties, concerns, distresses and diseases that come our way can be made more understandable and tolerable. At times we may even be able to remove some of the more straightforward difficulties we face by seeing them in a new light and so spotting a resolution, or a different approach that had not occurred to us before.

Holism or the holistic approach is not something new discovered in 1984. It has been written about in many different cultures using many different names over many centuries. We are only rediscovering what has been known before. What is new is that the basic assumptions or beliefs that underpin the holistic approach have, in the last seventy years, received the support of many eminent scientists and even more recently much medical research. So whereas before we might have had to possess a certain amount of faith to believe in the rudiments of a holistic approach, we can now draw on much that is modern and scientific – if we need to.

Historical perspective

From our very early beginnings on this planet, we have tried to make sense of our environment and our place on the cosmic stage. We started by believing we were insignificant and at the mercy of the gods. We created many different gods, each one carrying a particular power – wind, rain, fertility and so on – and we strove to appease and make sacrifices to these gods. Priests, witch-doctors and shamans became the mediators by which we could communicate with the gods. These early teachers were given special privileges and at times assumed the importance of gods in their own communities. Even though 'ordinary' people felt insignificant in relation to the gods, it was nevertheless believed that human beings and their world were important to the gods. Thus the earth was very much the centre of the universe and we were very much the chosen species that ruled over all other living creatures. For many hundreds of years these beliefs were firmly held. Illness and disease were seen as the result of some indiscretion committed in relation to one or other of the many gods. Sacrifice, prayer, ritual worship, laying on of hands, confession and penance were seen as the 'treatments' appropriate to afflicted individuals. Of course there were many exceptions to these approaches, but for a large part of our history much of the teaching about human origins and destiny was determined by the Church and its officers, from popes to priests. However, cracks slowly began to appear in the Church's universal hold on human society and the separation of Church and State that occurred in the fifteenth and sixteenth century signalled the 'rebirth' of man's progress, the renaissance.

By that time, Copernicus, the astronomer, had bravely published his life's work and put the sun at the centre of the universe, thus displacing the earth from its central position in the heavens. Galileo, who followed him, set about proving the brilliance of Copernicus' deductions, doing so with the aid of a giant telescope. So incensed were the elders of the Church at this 'blasphemous' behaviour that Galileo was arrested and, under pressure, recanted. The earth, however, did not return to the centre of the heavens and this progress in understanding ourselves and our world was unstoppable. The separation of religion from science had begun and was firmly encouraged by two other great scientists, Isaac Newton and René Descartes. Newton's view of the universe was governed by *reason* – all events took place as a result of mathematical laws which were determined by the principle law of cause and effect. He pointed out that gods and spirits had nothing to do with why we developed disease.

Newton's departure from old beliefs was further advanced by Descartes, who brought together and refined the principles which more or less guided the next 300 years of philosophical and scientific thought. Descartes, in one of his most famous observations, wrote, 'I think therefore I am'. By this statement not only did he help to separate the influence of gods and spirits from our mind, but he also separated the mind from the body. So although human beings were seen to comprise spirit, mind and body, each of these elements was seen to be separate and unconnected.

Descartes was not content with his philosophical thoughts. He went on to focus on the hard science of how the *body* functioned. He compared the workings of the body with those of a *clock*. He saw the body as a machine which worked because the parts within operated smoothly and mechanically. Descartes also went on to say how we should study the body to find out how it worked or did not work. Rather as with a machine, it was necessary 'to divide each of the difficulties into as many parts as possible and as might be necessary for its adequate solution'. Thus not only was the study of the body separated from the 'mind' and the 'spirit', but we were encouraged, as Francis Bacon wrote, to 'put the body on the rack and make it reveal its secrets'. What happened to the original teachers and healers of human distress? The priests were now confined to matters of the *spirit*. The barber surgeons and apothecaries took over the study of the *body*. The mind remained an enigma and no effective attempts to study how it worked were made until the studies of Freud late in the nineteenth century. The Church's influence was even further diminished through Darwin's discoveries and description of the evolution of the human species. No longer were we descendants of the inhabitants of the Garden of Eden: the human animal was nothing more than an evolved ape.

For the next few hundred years, after Descartes and Newton,

the study of the human condition, both healthy and diseased, was almost entirely in the hands of the 'doctor' as a scientist. The role of the doctor as a healer was inevitably less influential. Progress was apparent everywhere and by following Descartes' advice of reducing everything to its smallest part, Pasteur discovered bacteria and, it was thought, the causes of many human ills were finally understood. One bacterium caused one disease: the TB bacillus caused tuberculosis, the typhus bacillus caused typhus, and so on. Antibiotics heralded a major new development and now we not only understood what caused disease but could also pursue the medicines appropriate to each condition. Similarly, when vitamins were discovered, what could be clearer than that lack of vitamin C caused scurvy, lack of vitamin D caused rickets and so on?

Newton's notion of 'cause and effect' was beautifully illustrated, and any lingering ideas that the gods were involved in health and disease were swiftly banished. It was not only in medical treatment with the discovery of powerful drugs that progress was being made. With the development of safe anaesthetics and the sterile technique, surgeons were able to operate with improved results and with much less danger to the patient. In the mid-twentieth century, childbirth was no longer a potentially fatal condition and the survival rate amongst the new-born improved dramatically.

Several authors have argued that the progress in healthcare and longevity that occurred towards the beginning of the twentieth century was more the result of better housing and public health measures rather than the direct result of medical progress. They point out that over 90% of the total decline in mortality from such diseases as scarlet fever, cholera and tuberculosis occurred before immunisation and antibiotics were discovered. Nevertheless, the hold of science on medicine was by the beginning of the twentieth century almost total and the white-coat symbolised the new 'uniform' of the healer that contrasted starkly with the priest's robes and the witch-doctor's paint. Improved technology enabled doctors to probe into smaller and smaller portions of the human condition. The secrets of the cell were revealed and with the discovery of chromosomes, we progressed to the genetic theory and finally to the molecular theory of disease. More and more powerful drugs were developed and much of medical education was now given over to the learning of biochemistry and the study of neuropharmacology.

The criticisms of this *mechanistic* and *reductionistic* approach to the study of the human condition have always been present. William Blake parodied Newton's scientific method ('ration', as it was labelled) and illustrated it beautifully in his painting of God and of Newton measuring the universe with a compass. Blake also described one of the basic principles of what has since become known as a holistic perspective when he wrote these immortal words:

> To see a world in a grain of sand
> and a heaven in a wild flower,
> Hold infinity in the palm of your hand
> and eternity in an hour.
> Auguries of Innocence

In medicine as well, the doubters were always present. Even the great Pasteur, who is given credit for much of modern bacteriology, uttered the heretical words on his deathbed, 'The bacterium is nothing, the terrain is everything'.

Plato had once written:

> The cure of the part should not be attempted without treatment of the whole. No attempts should be made to cure the body without the soul, and if the head and body are to be healthy you must begin by curing the mind, for this is the great error of our day in the treatment of the human body that physicians first separate the soul from the body.

More recently, Hans Selye devoted his life to the understanding of *stress* or the syndrome of 'just being sick', as he first called it. His work, which spanned the greater part of this century, was a monument of deeper medical understanding. His approach to ill-health, beginning as it did from taking the whole person into account, was true to the holistic principle described by Blake – 'The whole is greater than the sum of its parts' and 'the part contains the whole'. As a result of Hans Selye's work, we now have a fairly good understanding as to how unhappiness can get into a cell, or how a difficult boss, or loss of a spouse, or bad living conditions, may play a part in the development of heart disease or cancer. Following his work, interested clinicians developed 'stress' clinics and were repeatedly finding that without recourse to drugs or surgery, many of the symptoms and signs of 'just being sick' could be reversed by using 'treatments' which focused on the *whole* person and not on the 'diseased' part.

Much of the remainder of this book is a description of the application of Selye's theories to the challenges of daily living. Selye's messages were not listened to by the majority of the medical profession and he was largely dismissed as an eccentric in his own lifetime. The criticisms, however, did not abate and in the last decade we have seen them increase to the point where the technological and scientific approach to medical care has found itself on the defensive.

Several authors stand apart in their well-reasoned arguments concerning the limitations of the reductionistic approach to medical care. Ivan Illich (who has combined the roles of parish priest in an Irish-Puerto Rican neighbourhood with that of a theologian, social thinker and agent provocateur of many professions) rocked the medical world with his book *Limits to Medicine*, or *Medical Nemesis* as it was first titled in 1976. His principal statement was that 'the medical establishment had become a major threat to health'. He outlined the epidemics of modern medicine and collected a large body of evidence to show how much of modern medical treatment is useless and potentially harmful. Amongst the many indictments were that:

(1) 15% of all hospital admissions are the result of medically-induced disease;
(2) 7% of all hospital admissions result in some compensatable injury.

He then went on to illustrate how the medical profession had influenced the health policies of various countries and had developed a stranglehold on how money was spent on health care and more importantly on *where* it was spent. He pointed out that because the medical profession was concerned with high technology and the scientific approach, a disproportionate part of our budget was spent on hospital-oriented services to the detriment of basic general practice and community services. The development of coronary care units and expenditure on high cost machines such as 'scans' and linear accelerators were a direct result of the medical profession's interests rather than because they benefited the consumer. We will come back to these points in later chapters.

Illich's most pungent criticisms against the medical profession were, however, levelled at the way it had influenced the belief-systems and values of the consumers. He felt that the 'promise' to end all pain and eliminate disease was a massive and tragic dehumanising confidence trick. Death can never be cheated and the medical profession's attempts to prolong life at all cost robbed man of his essential human existence. Illich saw the medicalisation of many of life's processes – birth, pregnancy, marriage, divorce, death – as an essentially anti-human act and put much of the blame on the medical profession's narrow and limited approach.

Illich's book was largely castigated in the medical press and his arguments, because they appeared so general and one-sided, were not taken very seriously. He failed to see how his case against the medical profession could not be separated from the ideology, culture and the society from which the medical profession arose. The collusion so apparent between doctors and patients was not sufficiently touched on and doctors were made the scapegoats of much that was wrong within their culture. It is important to understand how this 'collusion' prevents both doctor and patient from assuming their full potential. Achieving this potential involves an awareness of both the strengths and limitations present in each role. The doctor's ability to heal is influenced by the extent to which he is aware of the 'patient' within him. And the patient's ability to improve and get better is also influenced by the extent to which he is aware of the 'doctor' within him. What has happened in our culture is that all the 'healing powers' have been lodged in the doctor and all the 'illness' has been lodged in the patient. A holistic perspective involves letting go of this collusion and accepting a more participatory relationship between doctor and patient. The doctor lets go of his need for power and control and the patient lets go of his wish to be treated like a child and assumes some responsibility for his health.

In *The Role of Medicine* (1979) Thomas McKeown did not fall into that trap and although his own contributions support many of Illich's assertions, he distanced himself from many of the doctor-bashing remarks in *Limits to Medicine* and he says, 'The two books have little in common except perhaps in the sense that the Bible and the Koran could be said to be identified by the fact that both are concerned with religious matters'. His own viewpoint is to illustrate how 'for most diseases, prevention by control of their origins is cheaper, more humane, and more effective than intervention by treatment after they occur'.

McKeown uses a cultural, social and epidemiological 'pair of spectacles' to look at health and illness in our society. His views have been supported by many of the foremost social explorers of the nineteenth and twentieth century. Many of these reformers went to the very heart of the social and political divisions of our time. Class division, urban poverty, inequality in education, all play a part in determining the frequency and types of illness to which individuals are prone. Childbirth is a far more risky event for working-class wives than for middle-class women. More recently in the UK the Black Report (1982) has highlighted these inequalities in health in our own time.

Ian Kennedy in his book *The Unmasking of Medicine* (1981) describes some of the myths and fancies that surround the way in which medical decisions, both clinical and political, are made. He uses an 'ethical, legal and philosophical' pair of spectacles to look at the relationship between doctor and patient as well as medicine and society. He draws attention to the political nature of decisions surrounding the purchase of kidney machines, old people's homes and drug expenditure. Finally, Capra in his two books *The Tao of Physics* (1981) and *The Turning Point* (1983) completes the challenge to the reductionistic, mechanistic, dualistic notion of health and disease. Using the development of the 'new physics', he adds an up-to-date scientific explanation of the holistic approach. He draws on the discoveries of Einstein, Rutherford and Planck in the early part of this century and describes how the 'new physics' challenges the foundation of the Newtonian view of the universe. He writes: 'the new physics necessitated profound changes in concepts of space, time, matter, object and cause and effect'. 'Whereas in classical mechanics the properties and behaviour of the parts determine those of the whole, the situation is reversed in quantum mechanics: it is the *whole* that determines the behaviour of the parts.'

It is the application of this principle derived from 'quantum mechanics' that is the cornerstone of the holistic approach to health and disease. This revolutionary discovery in the most precise area of science can be applied to that most imprecise area 'human behaviour'. To the old Newtonian view of cause and effect is added the post-Einsteinian view of 'interpenetrating hierarchies' or systems theory.

It seems that what all these critics are saying can be summarised in the following propositions:

(1) Health is everyone's business and should not be left to the doctors.
(2) Health care involves ethical, moral and political decisions on the part of the planners and doctors.
(3) Patients should assume more responsibility for their own health care.
(4) Illness, diseases, pain, suffering and death are all part of the experience of being a human being and we cannot escape from these experiences.
(5) Promotion and preventive health care is cheaper, more effective and less dangerous than 'curative' and 'restorative' therapies. The meaning of an 'illness' may be sought on many different levels.
(6) Drugs and surgery do not allow us to care or even cure many of the current concerns of humankind.
(7) Low technology, primary health care delivered within the community should receive a higher priority than it now does.

The word 'holism' was first used by Smuts in 1928 in his book *Holism and Evolution*. He used it to describe the philosophical systems that looked on *whole* systems rather than parts. He suggested that it was as important to study how parts are connected with each other as it was to study the parts themselves. The word holism or holistic is derived from the Greek *holos* meaning 'whole', 'complete'. We derive our words 'hello' and 'health' from the same stem. The 'w' in 'wholism' is a recent addition to the spelling in the English language. How does this philosophical concept translate itself to the practical day-to-day issues of health and disease? Let us first try and expand a little on these concepts.

Body-mind-spirit

The human condition has, for the most part, been described as having three separate entities. Human beings have experienced themselves physically through the sensations – touch, sight, sound – as well as through the instincts of hunger, sex and self-preservation. We have experienced our minds through thoughts, ideas, concepts, images, and at times both body and mind are brought together through our emotions and feelings of anger, love, hate, compassion, in which both physical and psychological needs and perceptions are experienced. As we have seen, there has been a tendency to separate the body from the mind and to view each of the various aspects of the human condition as if it were able to exist independently of the others.

As we begin to discover the nature of the connection between mind and body, our level of *awareness* may change. In the same way as climbing a mountain will allow us to have a different perspective of the same view as we climb higher, so our greater awareness of the connectedness between body and mind will allow us to have a more complete 'view' of ourselves. When a climber is on the lower slopes of a mountain, the view he gets is 'true' only to a certain extent. The higher he gets, the clearer the view he can have of how illness in the individual is related to mental and social conditions. When doctors view the development of a stomach ulcer as a result of too much acid and treat the condition with antacids or by operation to stop the secretion of acid, their 'view' is solely based on a physical perspective. It is 'true', but only partly so. If they were to 'climb the mountain', they might see a different perspective which includes the physical one but begins to take into account the psychological one as well.

The man with a stomach ulcer may have thoughts, troubled thoughts. He may have feelings, anxious or frightened feelings. He may have a marriage that is in trouble or be about to be declared redundant. Personal factors and social conditions may all play their part. It is not that the 'ulcer' is all in his mind and that it is not real. The physicalness of his distress is as real as the mental symptoms he may or may not have. He may experience no mental distress and may well ask his doctor just to treat his ulcer and not ask too many questions about his sex-life. Both doctor and patient will then remain at the level of awareness they permit themselves to have. Like the mountain climber, they may not want to go on, it may be too dangerous. They are quite contented with the 'view' they already have and so on. Nevertheless, whether the doctor or patient proceeds, whether the mountain climber goes any further on, the 'view' is always there, even though no one may be there to observe it. What happens in the body is translated to the mind, and vice versa.

I suspect that for many people the connections between body and mind are relatively well-accepted, even if only to a small degree. What about the *spirit*? This is altogether different – this has to do with religions and faith, ritual and worship. No thoroughly modern scientist could accept a crude concept of spirit and, as we have seen, to accept a spiritual 'cause' to health and disease would be taking us back to the bad old days of witches and shamans' incantations and burning from which Descartes and Newton saved us in the seventeenth century. The notion of spirit or soul or 'driving force' need not of course be linked to religions or church-going. Just as it is possible to participate in a sport without belonging to a team or a sports club, so it is possible to have a spiritual experience without going to church. Pursuing the analogy of the mountain climber may allow us to explore how this 'experience' may be described.

He climbs this mountain and finally reaches the summit: sitting down, he pauses to look back at the climb and the view. His mind begins to wander and he finds he loses himself in the view – he begins to experience a sense of timelessness – he has been here all his life, yet in reality only a few minutes. The sense of who he is may vanish and he finds himself experiencing the trees or birds or clouds as if they were him, a feeling of connectedness/completeness or unity with all things which he finds impossible to describe may overwhelm him. He has the sense of having stumbled on the secrets of life and discovers that all that he experiences is there to be experienced. This mystical or spiritual state may occur for some whilst watching a play, or listening to music. It may occur whilst walking in the countryside or watching the ocean waves, making love, or watching a baby play.

It is best described by the poets and writers and here are a few examples of how such experiences have been described:

> . . . that serene and blessed mood
> In which the affections gently lead us on –
> Until, the breath of this corporeal frame
> And even the motion of our human blood
> Almost suspended, we are laid asleep
> In body, and become a living soul;
> While with an eye made quiet by the power
> of harmony, and the deep power of joy,
> We see into the life of all things.
> *Lines upon Tintern Abbey* by William Wordsworth

The thing happened one summer afternoon, on the school cricket field, while I was sitting on the grass, waiting my turn to bat. I was thinking about nothing in particular, merely enjoying the pleasures of midsummer idleness. Suddenly, and without warning, something invisible seemed to be drawn across the sky, transforming the world about me into a kind of tent of concentrated and enhanced significance. What had been merely an outside became an inside. The objective was somehow transformed into a completely subjective fact, which was experienced as 'mine', but on a level where the word had no meaning – for 'I' was no longer the familiar ego. Nothing more can be said about the experience, it brought no accession of knowledge about anything except, very obscurely, the knower and his way of knowing. After a few minutes there was a 'return to normalcy'. The event made a deep impression on me at the time; but, because it did not fit into any of the thought patterns – religious, philosophical, scientific – with which, as a boy of fifteen, I was familiar, it came to seem more and more anomalous, more and more irrelevant to 'real life', and was finally forgotten.

The Root of the Matter by Margaret Isherwood

Time present and time past
are both perhaps present in time future
and time future contained in time past.
If all time is eternally present
All time is unredeemable.

Burnt Norton by T. S. Eliot

These experiences have in common certain elements which lift them out of the ordinary emotional experiences one may have on a day-to-day basis. Their extra-ordinariness is often startling and for many they may mark the beginning of profound changes, psychological as well as physical. Although commonly described as 'religious experiences', they have been written about by many individuals who do not consider themselves to be religious. What is more, if one were to compare the descriptions of these 'mystical states' from different religions it is interesting to see how similar they are.

What these experiences attest to is that man has a capacity

to experience himself and the world about him in a way that is separate and different from the purely physical or psychological one. Whether we choose to exercise that capacity to have these experiences is another matter. Much like our climber on the mountain, we may choose to stop at a certain point. The view we then have of the world about us will be limited.

Let us go back to the man with his ulcer. We have seen how he can be treated on the physical level, with diet and antacids. We have seen how, if the doctor or patient chose to, the psychological level could be explored – his family life, work patterns etc. In what way might his 'ulcer' be explored from a 'spiritual perspective'? At first glance, it is difficult to see any connection and indeed it may be totally inappropriate for the doctor to suggest that there might be one. However, if the patient were to explore various questions – 'What *meaning* does this "ulcer" have for me?' 'What purpose is this ulcer serving?', 'Can I obtain a better picture (view?) of myself and my world having developed this ulcer?' – he may find that he quickly involves himself not in a physical or a psychological understanding but in a deeper level of 'knowing' which involves a more complete or 'holistic' appraisal of his situation. The ulcer may represent a 'hunger' for love; it may be the physical expression of some unexpressed longing, of some *thing* 'gnawing' at his life in general. At times the physicality of the symptoms or illness and the word or expressions we use may help us to identify a deeper level of meaning. We talk about 'shouldering a burden', 'broken-hearted', 'lump in our throat', 'tight-fisted'. Each of these phrases describes a state of mind or emotion which takes on a physical expression. Learning to translate our 'illnesses' into images or expressions of meaning may help us to understand their significance for our lives. It is this willingness to look for meaning and explore the connectedness of events that will allow for the 'spiritual' lessons that may require to be learned.

Quite rightly for the majority of us, the physical level of understanding of disease is often as far as we wish to go. But a truly 'holistic' approach may require both doctor and patient to involve themselves in a much more prolonged and complex exploration.

Families

As individuals, of course, we are only a 'part of a great whole'. Each individual was and is part of a 'family'. The family unit may vary from an extended family with grandparents and cousins, to a nuclear family consisting of husband, wife and children or a single-parent family. Some of us may not feel part of a family at all and our 'illness' may well stem from that fact. Much has been written about the break-up of the traditional family and the impact this has had on the health of individuals. Levels of stress and depression can often be linked to family disturbances. The loss of a husband or wife may lead to some form of illness in the survivor. Loneliness, isolation and alienation, often consequences of fractured families, are common precursors of both psychological as well as physical illnesses. Obtaining support from other members of our family may help us to recover and at times actually to survive an illness. Sometimes families 'need' someone to be the invalid as a way of holding it together. Young children are often taken to a doctor as a symptom of some marital difficulty between husband and wife. Thus when trying to understand a particular symptom of illness from a holistic perspective, it may be necessary to look at the family from which that individual arises or in which he or she currently resides.

Community

The family itself is also part of a greater 'whole'. The neighbourhood or community does have an impact on the family. An Asian family living in the East End of London may feel threatened to such an extent that it ceases to function as a unit, which in turn puts a greater strain on the individuals within it, which in turn leads to physical or psychological dis-ease. Conversely, a well-knit community, as found in some of the villages in South Wales or Yorkshire, can support and give sustenance to families under pressure and economic hardship, as happened only recently in the miners' strike. Indeed the external pressure may help to bring families and individuals closer together, and this closeness may go a long way to prevent and, at times, actually reduce the onset of disease. A community that takes pride in its environment, that looks after its natural resources, that is open to changes but remains true to its fundamental values, acts as a large 'family' for the smaller individual 'families' within it.

A survey done in a London housing estate identified households whose levels of 'health' were very much higher than the average household. Individuals within such households had less 'illness', described themselves as happy and fulfilled, made fewer visits to doctors etc. What was interesting and surprising was that these households were surrounded by other households with increasing levels of good health. In other words, the health of these families was 'infectious' to their neighbours. The idea that 'health' as well as 'disease' is infectious is very much part of a holistic approach. Seeking out 'healthy', 'alive' and 'joyful' people may be a necessary part of a recovery process or convalescence.

Nation

Communities may not have that much freedom in determining their environment. Levels of taxation are determined by central government. Policies on health-care provision and such matters as pollution, tobacco, taxation, food policies, fluoridation, are not determined at an individual, family or community level, yet they have a large impact on health. Indeed the major threat to our health comes from the decisions central government makes over such issues as the defence of the nation and the potential use of nuclear weapons. Thus we see again how communities are only part of a greater 'whole', and how that *'whole' has an influence on the health of the part*. This is one of the fundamental principles of the holistic approach and is best illustrated by this story:

> 'What is Fate?' Nasruddin was asked by a scholar.
> 'An endless succession of intertwined events each influencing each other.'
> 'That is hardly a satisfactory answer – I believe in cause and effect.'
> 'Very well,' said the Mullah. 'Look at that.' He pointed to a procession passing in the street. 'That man is being taken to be hanged. Is that because someone gave him a silver piece and enabled him to buy the knife with which he committed murder, or because someone saw him do it, or because nobody stopped him?'

This principle takes us away from the simple notion that a 'disease' has either a simple cause or that it can be 'cured' by suppressing the symptoms or cutting out the diseased part. These approaches, which are undoubtedly effective on occasion for treatment, do not necessarily bring about a cure. For disease can now be seen as an imbalance between the 'parts' and the 'whole' and 'cures' may rarely, if ever, be possible. Nevertheless, by looking at the *connections* between the parts and the *whole* as well as the connections between the *whole* and the parts, we may begin to get an idea as to how true healing can occur. We shall start by using the concept of stress to describe this imbalance between parts and whole.

2

STRESS – AN IMBALANCE BETWEEN PARTS AND THE WHOLE

There is a lot of confusion over the word 'stress'. Most of us have some understanding of what it means to us personally and how it affects us. Scientists, psychologists and doctors all have different definitions. In the medical world, although stress is recognised as a major causative factor in many conditions, the word stress is not in favour. It is not precise enough and we have difficulty in measuring it accurately, unlike blood counts or heart rates.

Nevertheless, stress is central to our discussion and we shall need to define it. Hans Selye, who was the pioneer of modern stress work, used to define it as the 'syndrome of just being sick'. That, however, was not scientific enough for his colleagues and he went on to use the following definition: 'The state manifested by a specific syndrome which consists of all the non-specifically induced changes within a biological system'. The first definition appears more understandable and it may be easier to describe the way we shall use stress by saying what stress is not.

Stress is not simply nervous tension;
is not just an emergency release of adrenalin;
is not necessarily something bad;
cannot and should not be avoided;
can result from positive (happy) as well as negative (bad) changes.

Stress can be seen as a very necessary part of life: it can be seen as a sign that we are out of balance in some way with ourselves and our environment. If we remain out of balance for long we may move into a 'stressed state' which, as we shall see, has different ways of showing itself for each of us. 'Stress' results as part of the process of responding to changes that occur both within ourselves (thoughts, feelings, food, breathing

17

pattern) as well as outside ourselves (friends, work, noise, atmospheric pollution). As a change occurs in our lives and we respond to it, we alter in some way our physical or psychological experience, e.g. our heart may have to beat faster, our thoughts or feelings are altered, we change and produce an imbalance, which may be temporary, in ourselves. Let me give you an example of how both a 'positive' as well as 'negative' change can bring about an imbalance and 'stress'.

Imagine an office worker during the Second World War returning home one evening after a busy day. She goes into her kitchen to make herself a cup of tea and takes it into the front room, takes off her shoes and puts her feet up. The door bell rings, she goes to the door with the cup of tea in her hand, opens it and there stands a policeman with a message from the Ministry of Defence. Her son, serving in France, has been reported killed in action. She drops her cup, screams out aloud, starts shaking and crying, her heart beats faster and her breathing becomes erratic. She may even faint. Now imagine this lady four years later. She has adjusted to the death of her son. She is again returning from work, makes herself a cup of tea and is ready to relax when the door bell rings. Another policeman with another message – her son has after all been discovered in a POW camp and is alive and well. She drops her cup again, screams out aloud, bursts into tears, her heart beats faster and her breathing becomes erratic.

Two totally different messages, one negative and one positive, producing almost exactly the same response and bringing about a 'state of imbalance' or 'stress' in the same individual. If that state of imbalance were allowed to continue, then the individual might show signs of a *stressed state*. The response to the change is not in itself 'bad' or 'wrong' – i.e. stress cannot be avoided, it is part of life.

It may help at this stage to introduce a few more definitions. Selye coined the word *stressor* to describe the changes in our internal or external world, e.g. noise, change of job, food. A *stressor* is the agent that makes a demand on the individual and produces a change or response which results in a state of imbalance, however temporary. This response Selye called a *stress-response*.

To appreciate this acceleration of change, it is helpful to see progress in the last hundred years against the perspective of the history of our universe and formation of the earth.

Our present time perspective

Big Bang (formation of universe)		1 January
Formation of Earth		14 September
Origin of life		25 September
Significant oxygen		1 December
First fish		19 December
First mammals		26 December
First humans		31 December
First cave painting	11.59 pm	31 December
Christ	11.59.56 pm	
Renaissance	11.59.59	
Present day	First second of New Year's Day	

Many of the changes are obvious to see – the rapid growth of population (world population is doubling every 11 years). Half the energy used by man in the last 2000 years has been consumed in the last 100 years. The 'life' of our electrical appliances is on average 5–7 years, whereas it was 20 years from the 1900s to the 1940s. Even the teddy bears and dolls we give our children do not last them the same length of time. We have a new house, job, marriage more often than we did 40 years ago. We are overwhelmed with information overload (90% of all scientists that ever lived are alive today). In 1500, books were being printed at the rate of 1000 a year. In 1980 this figure was 1000 new books a day.

We can illustrate this model of understanding stress by the following diagram:

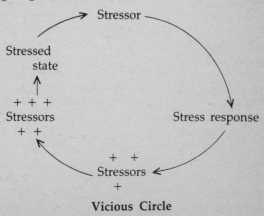

Vicious Circle

19

The *stressed state* is the result of an accumulation of *stress responses* which occur as a result of numerous stressors. As we shall see, the stressed state is different for different individuals and we each have our own individual patterns of stress response.

One of the reasons why the *stressed state* is thought to be more common in the modern twentieth-century Western world is that there appear to be many more *stressors* or changes that we have to negotiate with. Alvin Toffler in his book *Future Shock* gives some graphic examples of how the number of 'changes' or pace of life has increased.

This increase in 'pace' means we have many more stressors and one of the reasons people seek to 'drop out' or go to live in the country and start farming or living in a commune is that it is seen as a way of decreasing the number of stressors. Holidays, which are the more normal way of decreasing stressors, often begin and end with increasing demands of passport control, luggage and customs inspection. New faces, new hotels etc. are all *stressors* demanding *stress response*. It is no wonder that it takes a few days before some people fully unwind and return to a 'state of balance'. We can now see why a wedding, a presumably 'happy' change, can become, and is for some, a stressful event. There are a cluster of stressors all occurring at once. A marriage involves a possible change of work, and home, diet patterns and sleeping patterns may all change. The demands of a change in sexual activity all bring about increased stress responses and the potential for stressed state. We now need to describe the stress response in some more detail if we are to understand why new marriages do not collapse after the third week.

Stress response

The 'stress response' is the response made by an individual to a stressor. If the telephone rings whilst I am busy with some other activity, it acts as a stressor, a change. I may respond with irritation, the *fight response*, or I may choose to ignore it and continue with what I am doing, the *flight response*, or I may decide to *flow* with the stressor and accept the interruption with some tolerance and equanimity, or, as Robert Elliott has put it, 'If you can't fight or flee, then flow'. These stress responses describe the way in which the majority of us act in a variety of different situations. The same stressor can cause different stress responses in different individuals, and similarly, each individual can respond to the same stressor differently. Let us look at each stress response in some detail. We shall describe the 'extreme' of each response to highlight its features.

Fight response

(a) The *external fight* response is characteristic of the highly competitive, energetic individual. He or she has a tendency to quantify achievements rather than to enjoy them. They are impatient, always with a sense of time pressure, moving on to the next demand before the previous one is met. They are workaholics and have difficulty in relaxing. At their worst, they are aggressive, irritable and overbearing. They are high achievers and often do not suffer fools gladly. Someone who constantly uses a 'fight response' to stressors has been described as having the 'A' type personality. Many individuals who use a fight response are, of course, not necessarily that extreme, but the constant use of the fight response has a tendency to develop the personality in that direction. The over-use of this response may also lead to physical disorders and it is classically associated with heart disease, especially coronary disease.

(b) *The internal fight response* – here the individual, although responding with a fight response, does not express it externally, but rather gives the impression of being 'in control'. They tend to be orderly, tidy, precise and consistent. They appear unemotional and at their worst become obsessional and repetitive in both their thoughts and actions. Again, this is an extreme description, and on many occasions it is appropriate to adopt an 'internal fight' response to stressors. However, individuals who consistently use this response may develop a tendency towards gastro-intestinal disease such as peptic ulcers, or the equally common, irritable bowel syndrome. At this stage, it should be emphasised that it is not that a particular stress response is 'good' or 'bad'. It is more important for us to be able to use each of the stress responses in different situations as appropriate. It is the over-use of some particular response to whatever the stressor that leads to a fixed and rigid pattern and eventually a stressed state.

21

Flight response

Here the response is usually to avoid the stressor; the unpaid bill is forgotten, the opportunity for advancement is turned down. Such individuals are cautious and conservative. They appear vulnerable and dependent. They are unassertive and under-achievers. They feel at the 'mercy of the world' and can withdraw into their own 'private' self where they remain aloof, isolated and suspicious. The constant use of the flight response is associated with the 'phobic personality' or the despair syndrome which recently has been linked to the development of certain types of cancer. Again, it is important to emphasise that the *flight response* may be perfectly appropriate in certain situations, e.g. major external threat, fire or overwhelming stressors, but the constant over-use of this response will lead to as many psychological and physical problems as will the fight response.

The fight and flight responses are very much ingrained within our biological system. For many thousands of years when man was living in the jungles and primitive inimical environments, these responses were more than adequate for the stressors he was likely to meet. However, as man has become more urbanised, socialised and civilised, the fight and flight responses are not always the most appropriate ones for him to adopt. He has had to develop and use a third response called the 'flow response'.

Flow response

This response can be described as a 'merging' or flowing with the stressor of the moment. 'Stay cool', the universal expression of the 1960s generation, captures the quality of the response. Neither a fight nor a flight, the individual is responsive and tolerant to the change in the environment. At first glance, this response may appear to be always preferable to the previous two. However, individuals who consistently use this response may appear changeable and erratic. They appear to be inconsistent, having no firm sense of values or beliefs. Because they neither fight nor flee, they may develop a sense of not belonging; nothing matters other than their own self-survival. The me-too or narcissistic generation belong to this group who constantly use the flow response. 'Anything goes' means they develop frequent minor illnesses or accidents. They are obsessed with their health and seek out any new health fad that is around. They chase the flavour of the month and appear to lack any firm conviction in anything. Because of this tendency to flow they are prone to the charismatic leader and join cults or religious sects, flowing with the strong pull of the guru.

Again, it is important to emphasise that it is the over-use of one response to whatever the stressor that develops into this fixed, mental and physical pattern. Although we each of us have our own preferred response, we can, with practice, begin to choose between the responses. It is important for us to be able to use each of the stress responses in different situations as appropriate. The over-use of one stress response or repeated mismatching of stress response to stressor is likely to lead to a stressed state of ill-health.

> **Exercise I**
> Identify a stressor that is likely to occur in the next week, e.g. a demand at work, or a chore at home. Identify your usual stress response – is it *fight*, *flight* or *flow*? Make a conscious decision to alter your usual response to this impending stressor. If you normally use a fight response, adopt a flight or flow response and observe what happens. Choose a stressor that is not too important. Do not try to fly before you can walk.

Look back at the diagram on page 19. We have discussed stressors and stress response. Now we will examine the stressed state and see how we can tell that we are in it.

Stressed state – warning signs – symptoms

Before we discuss these in detail, it is important to return to our concept of holism and describe another, second important principle. As we have seen, the human being has a physical, psychological and spiritual experience both of himself and his external world. These aspects of ourselves do not act separately and independently. They are all interrelated and interconnected. What happens in the body affects the mind and what happens in the mind affects the body. It is not that our physical symptoms or diseases are 'all in the mind'. It is that the mind, the seat of thoughts, ideas, emotions, fantasies and hopes, finds expression through the body, and the body involving itself in breathing, walking, eating, relaxing and exercise etc. affects the quality of our thoughts, ideas, hopes, etc. How our 'spiritual awareness' affects us is not so clear but we shall attempt to describe that later on.

One of the most important principles of holism and indeed stress management to grasp is the *interrelatedness and interconnectedness of body-mind-spirit*. Imagine that we develop a warning sign of a stressed state – e.g. a headache: something indeed may be wrong with our head – tense muscles, dilated arteries – but it is important to find out whether the headache has arisen from some troubled or anxious thoughts. Similarly, if we find ourselves feeling anxious or troubled, it is important to find out whether a poor posture or something in the diet has been the cause. Equally important is the awareness that it may be a combination of factors. A holistic approach requires a holistic outlook.

(1) Muscular system – Symptoms connected with this system are the most common and they result from an increase in muscular tension. Symptoms may be felt anywhere in the body, but usually the *back of the neck or lower back* is the first area. *Headaches* are the result of increased tension of the muscles, at times accompanied by feelings of *nausea or sickness*. Tension in the *jaw muscles* leads to *grinding of teeth* and can produce an imbalance in *alignment of the spine*. Tightening of the muscles of the face leads to pain over the *eyes and forehead*. Any of the muscles in the body can be affected and some do not produce any obvious symptom like pain or tension. The most common groups of muscles to be so affected are the *diaphragm*, which is a dome-shaped muscle separating the contents of the abdomen from the chest, and the *pelvic muscles* deep in the lower part of the abdomen surrounding the sexual organs.

Increased tension of the *throat muscles* can lead to the sensation of a 'lump in the throat', can affect speech, and accounts, in part, for the *high-pitched* and *nervous laughter* not uncommonly found in people under tension.

If the muscular tension is severe, then it can lead to *trembling, shaking, nervous tics,* or frequent *blinking*. If any 'warning sign' of a stressed state is not attended to, it can produce not only short-term discomfort but long-term disability and disease. In addition to the muscles that help us move and are under our conscious control, there is a group of muscles known as *involuntary muscles* surrounding blood vessels and the intestines which in turn are also affected by the stressed state and produce a whole variety of 'warning signs', some only apparent to the doctor on examination, others causing troublesome symptoms for those individuals affected. These include:

(a) *Raised blood pressure* because of 'tension' in the muscles surrounding the arteries.

(b) *Migraine headaches* – the muscles surrounding the arteries of the scalp first constrict (tighten) then dilate (expand), giving rise to the throbbing one-sided headache.

(c) *Intestinal symptoms* from *'rumbling of the stomach'* to *'burping'* or *increase in flatus.* The 'irritable bowel syndrome' which causes *intermittent diarrhoea* and *constipation* and is often associated with *pain* and *distension of the abdomen* results from a disturbance in the muscle tone surrounding the lower gut. These symptoms are also accompanied by loss of appetite.

(2) Glandular system – the stressed state may result in many disturbances of the different glands in the body, the most frequent and obvious being *excessive sweating*, resulting in *damp palms* and *unpleasant smell*. Similarly, *dryness* of the *throat and mouth* with *difficulty in swallowing* is a common symptom for some individuals.

(3) Heart and lungs – rapid pulse rate, pounding of the heart, palpitations, rapid shallow breathing or overbreathing known as hyperventilation, are common warning signs of someone in a stressed state.

(4) Nervous system – dizziness, fainting spells and general feeling of weakness and lethargy can develop into loss of 'joie de vivre' and affect sleep. Difficulty in getting off to sleep as well as waking up early and tired are very common warning signs. Not so well recognised but equally common is sleeping too much. Sleep which is disturbed by dreams or nightmares is frequent for those individuals who are possibly repressing some conscious thoughts during the day. The way we can use dreams to help us understand ourselves and the function they serve in keeping us balanced will be described later in Chapter 7 (pages 113ff.).

(5) Mind – general warning signs

(a) Inability to concentrate – not being able to focus on anything for long.

(b) General irritability or overexactingness which is often followed by periods of sadness, lethargy and depression.

(c) *Floating anxiety* – having a sense of mild fear or panic but not quite knowing why.

On occasions, the mind is unsettled or distressed: the only way that we can recognise this to be so, is by observing our *behaviour* or *habits*. Obvious habits such as *excessive smoking* or *drinking* and *increased use of tranquillisers* or food bingeing are easy to identify. Other behaviours or habits equally destructive may include promiscuous sexual activity or accident proneness.

It is possible to expand this list indefinitely, but what is more helpful is that each of us should become aware of our own 'warning signs'. They serve to tell us that we are in the stressed state – similar to the red light that goes on on the dashboard to indicate that the car has run out of oil. Unfortunately, what tends to happen is that we ignore the red light or we divert our attention to something else. What is worse is when we visit our doctor and his approach is to give a drug or treatment that only helps to 'knock the red light out'. These warning signs are invaluable markers and guides that let us know we are in a state of imbalance either with ourselves or our environment. By all means find something to relieve the distress or pain, but make sure it is something that helps in returning you to a state of balance and not something which affects the warning sign only.

Exercise II

On a sheet of paper put the headings

Body   *Mind* – thoughts   *Feelings*   *Behaviour*

and list all the warning signs with which you are familiar. Ask a close friend, husband or wife to indicate those warning signs with which you may not be familiar.

So far in this chapter we have looked at the three elements in the diagram on page 19 – the vicious circle. The three elements are *stressors*, *stress responses* and *stressed state*. In the descriptions of these three elements, we have tried to raise our *awareness* as to the content of the elements and we can now begin to describe how we can bring about some changes. *Awareness*, however, is the clue to most of the subsequent work.

If we are not aware of our stressors or patterns of stress responses or, even worse, the warning signs of the stressed state, then there is little we can do to bring about change.

When we were describing the holistic approach, an emphasis was made on the *connectedness* and interrelatedness between *parts* and *whole*. Increasing our awareness of the parts (BODY-MIND-SPIRIT-FAMILY etc.) will allow us to become aware of their interconnectedness. Self-awareness is not the same as self-centredness or narcissistic preoccupation. Building up one's awareness of the parts of oneself allows for a greater awareness of the parts of others and gives us a freedom of choice we otherwise would not have.

To turn the vicious circle into a benign circle we need to intersperse a new element into it. This new element we shall call the *holistic response*.

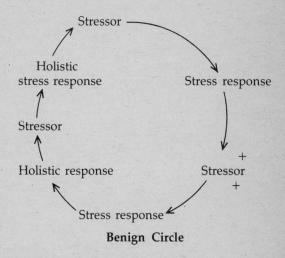

Benign Circle

The holistic response

The holistic response is the phrase we shall use to describe a series of approaches, coping-skills, stress-management techniques, exercise routines, good habit patterns, that will help to undo the stressed state and bring the body-mind-spirit complex back into a state of balance. These will now be listed and described in some more detail in subsequent chapters.

The holistic response
* increasing awareness
* taking responsibility in self-care
* finding an appropriate balance between opposite tensions
* developing a personal life-plan

* creating a personal and social support system
* practising specific coping skills
  breathing and relaxation techniques
      allowing time for silence and meditation
      exercise routine
      letting go
      creative visualisation
* attention to diet and nutrition
* developing communication skills

It is obvious from the list above that there is more than one life-time's work involved in the 'holistic response'. No one individual could hope to be able to learn or put into practice all these activities. Nevertheless, one of the characteristics of individuals who are effective at managing stress in general is that they have a repertoire of approaches which permits choice and gives them the sense of being in control of their lives. As you learn about some of these suggestions, some will appeal to you and you will be able to use them almost at once. Others you will find more difficult and they may require some practice, and even then you may not find them helpful. Try and at least work through each of the suggestions before you decide they are not for you.

3

UNDER-STANDING HOW TO RELAX YOUR BODY

The ancient philosophers used to say the body was like 'The Temple of God'. It was necessary to keep the temple clean, peaceful and well-attended so that one might hear the voice of God more clearly. We do not need to accept this exact comparison to appreciate that our bodies require to be looked after if our minds and spirit are to function well. It is worth repeating that understanding how the body-mind-spirit are interconnected is one of the fundamental principles of the holistic approach.

The important areas that we shall discuss in this and subsequent chapters have to do with those functions of the body that are specifically related to the stressed state. Rather than describe the body as if it were just a machine, with different moving parts, we shall outline some of the everyday activities we do with our bodies, with the intention of increasing your awareness of these activities. Several exercises will be described which will allow you to take some control over the way the body responds to the stressed state.

Breathing

Breathing is the most important and vital act we do. We rarely give much thought to how we breathe. If we stop breathing, we die, and we recognise this fact in our language when we talk about someone 'expiring' and conversely we talk about being 'inspired' and taking a 'good breath in' as ways of achieving positive health. Most of us recognise that our breathing alters in pattern and rhythm throughout the day. How that breathing alters may be influenced by how we feel. Again we talk about 'gasping for breath' or 'catching one's breath' or we say that something 'took my breath away'. We may also be aware of how our breathing increases when we get excited or how we sigh when we are sad or depressed. On occasions we may stop breathing altogether for as much as half a minute, and it is not uncommon for some children to have breath-holding attacks which are often associated with anger and temper tantrums.

One other most important fact about breathing is that it can take place without our thinking about it and also that we can alter it at will. We can slow down or increase our breathing if we choose to. It is one of the very few activities of the body in which there is both conscious control and automative activity. This breathing forms a link between the conscious and unconscious parts of our being. By observing and increasing the awareness of our breathing we can obtain useful information as to how our whole being is operating. Breathing is the most sensitive indicator or warning sign that we possess. Consciously increasing one's awareness about breathing and practising some of the breathing exercises we shall describe can be the most important steps anyone can take to improve their well-being, decrease the level of stress and help to bring about a sense of the interconnections between body, mind and spirit.

How do we breathe?

Breathing is the activity that brings oxygen from the atmosphere into the lungs and expels carbon dioxide and other waste products from the lungs into the atmosphere. The lungs are situated in the chest, covered by a thin but tough layer called the pleura, and surrounded by the ribs and muscles of respiration. The muscles of respiration are of three types:

(1) **(Inter)-Costal muscles**
Muscles between the ribs on the chest wall.

(2) **Diaphragm**
Dome-shaped muscle separating the chest cavity from the abdominal contents.

(3) **Accessory muscles of respiration**
These are situated at the top end of the rib cage together with some muscles of the back and abdomen.

Chest breathing

This is characterised by an upward and outward movement of the chest due to contraction of the costal (rib) muscles. This type of breathing is found most typically during vigorous exercise or in emergency situations. It allows the chest to expand quickly and is the most efficient way of obtaining oxygen quickly. Chest breathing may also help to arouse us and you may find yourself taking a deep breath and expanding your chest when you first wake up. Using the costal muscles for breathing, however, is not the 'normal' or 'natural' way for us to breathe during other situations not associated with exercise or arousal. Even so, what has happened for many individuals is that they maintain a costal pattern of breathing even following the cessation of the emergency situation. A constant use of chest breathing keeps the body in a state of constant arousal and the body acts as if it is experiencing a stressor. Let me give you an illustration.

Imagine you are driving a car and suddenly a small child runs across the road. Your immediate reaction is to slam on the brakes, grip the steering wheel, tighten your muscles, breathe more rapidly with an exaggerated inspiration or gasp. You just miss the child and start accelerating again. You may breathe a sigh of relief – breathing out forcefully – and relax your grip on the steering wheel. What may happen, however, and what often does happen, is that you may maintain your high state of arousal: you still continue to breathe shallowly with your chest muscles and you still maintain your increased muscle tension. In other words, you maintain your stress response for much longer than is appropriate. Your body has not returned to a state of balance and you will have to respond to your next stressor from a position of heightened state of arousal. Learning to let go and release the tension accumulated as a result of your stress response is essential if you are to avoid the stressed state.

The clue as to how to do this was given in the example and can be better understood after we have described the second way in which we breathe.

Diaphragmatic Breathing

The diaphragm is a horizontal dome-shaped muscle which separates the contents of your chest (heart and lungs) from your abdomen (stomach, liver, intestines). On inspiration, the diaphragm contracts, flattens and descends, thus creating a 'vacuum' in the chest, and air is sucked in. As the diaphragm descends it pushes the abdominal contents down and the increase in pressure forces the abdominal wall (the front of your abdomen) out. On expiration, the diaphragm relaxes and forces air out of the lungs, reducing the pressure on the abdominal contents and causing the abdominal wall to flatten.

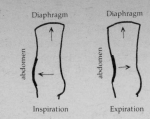

Figure 4

Diaphragm   Diaphragm

abdomen   abdomen

Inspiration   Expiration

It is important to note that the abdominal muscles do not normally contract during diaphragmatic breathing – they only respond passively to the increase in pressure in the abdomen. If you watch a small baby breathing you will see its abdomen moving up and down. The baby is breathing with its diaphragm, which is the normal and healthy way to breathe. When the baby cries or is hungry or distressed, the pattern of its breathing will change to a chest or costal rhythm. Unfortunately this pattern of breathing is encouraged by such statements as 'stick your chest out when you breathe' or 'flatten your stomach'. Thus we develop a chronic pattern of rapid shallow chest breathing during childhood and into adulthood and consider this pattern to be normal – it may be 'normal' but it is certainly unhealthy.

Diaphragmatic breathing requires less 'energy' than chest breathing: it allows for expansion of the bases of the lungs and the up and down motion of the diaphragm gently massages the abdominal organs. Chronic chest breathers breathe 12–16 full breaths a minute whereas regular diaphragmatic breathing requires only 8–10 breaths a minute. This works out at 16,000–18,000 breaths a day in chest breathing as opposed to 8,000–11,000 in diaphragmatic breathing. Over a lifetime of breathing this can amount to a large difference in energy expanded. However, probably the most important difference, as has been mentioned already, is that chronic chest breathing keeps the body and mind in a chronic state of arousal.

Mouth/nose breathing

Most of us naturally breathe through our nostrils and we are all aware of what a discomfort it is when we cannot, either because we have a cold or an allergy. It is important in the breathing cycle for other reasons as well. The air is warmed and moistened in the nose before entering the lungs, but more importantly the air stimulates delicate nerve endings in the lining of the nose which serve to reduce the level of arousal present in the body and so help to calm the mind. Snoring and breath apnoea (periods of breath holding) are associated with chronic mouth breathing and may lead to disturbances in the sensitive auto-nomic-nervous system which will be described later on.

Inhalation/exhalation

The breath cycle consists of inhalation and exhalation. When we were children no one told us whether we should pause between breaths or not. Recent medical discoveries, however, have begun to link some disturbances of breathing rhythm and pattern with specific medical conditions. Breathing retraining programmes are being introduced in several medical centres dealing with coronary disease, high blood pressure and chronic lung conditions. The 'hyperventilation syndrome' (breathing pattern of rapid shallow chest breathing) accounts for many strange presentations to doctors – dizziness, chest pains, migraine, cramps, 'nervousness', phobias, etc. What we do know is that retraining individuals to breathe through their *nostrils* with their *diaphragm* in regular, even, rhythmical patterns where the inhalation is as long as the exhalation and there is little or no pause between inhalation and exhalation produces immediate benefit for the majority of patients in reducing their arousal level and long-term benefits in a substantial proportion of patients in undoing the effects of a chronic state of arousal.

Try it and see for yourself

Exercise I – Relaxation Response

Find a quiet room where you will be undisturbed for about 10–15 minutes. Lie down on the bed or floor. Undo any tight clothing and remove your shoes. Spend a few moments settling yourself down. Close your eyes, spread your feet 12–18 inches apart and check that your head, neck and spine are in a straight line. Now focus your attention on your breathing. Do not try and change your breathing for the moment. Become aware of how fast or slow you are breathing, whether you are breathing with your chest or diaphragm. Notice whether there are any gaps or pauses between your inhalation and exhalation. – *Pause* – Now put one hand on your upper chest and one hand on your abdomen just below your rib-cage. Relax the shoulders and hands. As you exhale allow the abdomen to flatten. There should be little or no movement in the chest. Allow yourself a little time to get into a regular rhythm – *Pause* – It may help to imagine that as you are breathing in, you draw half a circle with your breath and as you breathe out, you complete the second half of the circle. – *Pause* – Allow your breath to become smooth, easy and regular. – *Pause* – Now consciously slow down your exhalation and allow your inhalation to follow smoothly and easily. – *Pause* – smooth out any gaps or pauses in your breathing. – *Pause* – if any distractions, thoughts or worries come into your mind, allow them to come, then allow them to go and bring your attention back to your breathing. – *Pause* – When you are ready to end this exercise, take a few deeper breaths in. Bring some feeling back into your fingers and toes. Open your eyes slowly and turn over on to one side before gently sitting up.

This exercise has been practised by Yogis over thousands of years to help them quieten their bodies and minds. Howard Benson, an American cardiologist, introduced it to his heart patients and called it the Relaxation Response. Dr Patel, a general practitioner in Croydon, has developed this exercise for her patients with high blood pressure. It is similar to exercises used in natural childbirth classes and has also been used to help people with sleeping problems or people wanting to come off tranquillisers. The idea that we need to learn how to breathe to remain healthy and relaxed may appear very strange at first but countless patients and doctors are learning to breathe with their diaphragms for the first time for many years and are helping to undo the effects of chronic stress patterns. Try and get into the habit of spending at least ten minutes a day breathing this way. It is not essential for you to lie on the floor or bed, and you can practise your breathing waiting in a traffic jam or sitting on a bus. The important thing is to begin increasing your awareness of your own breathing pattern and take some control over it.

This can be encouraged by reminding yourself to check your breathing during the course of the day. Stop for a few moments wherever you are and check to see whether you are breathing with your chest muscles or diaphragm. Check to see whether you stop breathing – this is especially common whilst answering the telephone. Gradually build up your awareness of your breathing pattern until you no longer are awkward about doing it.

Muscle tension and progressive relaxation

Next to altered and unhealthy breathing patterns, the stressed state affects the muscles of the body. In the last chapter we indicated certain groups of muscles that were commonly affected and it will now be important to describe these groups in some more detail. Muscles get tense (contract) during a stress response because of an increase in nervous stimulation. Nerves carry the message from the brain to all the different muscle groups in the body and also carry back messages from the muscle groups to the brain. By relaxing the muscles we reduce the 'messages' carried back to the brain and help to free energy for other activity. Here is another example of the body-mind-body-mind link. Muscles are of two types – the voluntary and involuntary muscles. It is with the voluntary muscles we are concerned at present.

VOLUNTARY MUSCLES	SYMPTOMS PRODUCED BY TENSION	INVOLUN-TARY MUSCLES	SYMPTOMS PRODUCED BY TENSION
Eye	Eye strain	Around arteries	High blood pressure
Back of Neck	Tension headache	Around bowel	Irritable bowel syndrome (constipation/diarrhoea)
Back	Back pain	Around stomach	Passing wind

There have been several approaches described to help people relax – they all have in common the instruction of 'letting go'. Telling people to relax can often make them more tense and one of the earlier books on this subject was called *You Must Relax* –

not a very conducive title. Some people are also not aware of when their muscles are tense and when they are relaxed. Again we see how the word awareness is mentioned. The best way of finding out whether your muscles are tense or relaxed is to increase the tension, which we can do much more easily than relaxing and then 'letting go' the tension. When we let go, the muscles return to a more relaxed state than they were in before we increased the tension. Also the process of 'letting go' is easier to learn from your 'increased tense' state than from 'normal' state.

Exercise II
Find a quiet room where you will be undisturbed for 10–15 minutes. Remove your shoes and loosen any tight clothing. You can do this exercise sitting, but it is preferable to lie down on a bed or carpet. Close your eyes gently – make sure your head, neck and trunk are straight.

Start by raising your eyebrows and tensing the muscles of your forehead. Keep the tension counting to five – then relax the muscles and become aware of any difference you feel in the muscles. Repeat once more. Now squeeze your eyes as tight as you can, forcing your eyes shut. Count to five, then release. Notice any difference. Repeat once more. Open your mouth wide, stretching the muscles of your face to the centre of the face, puckering up your lips, eyebrows and chin. Count to five – release – repeat once more. Tighten the muscles of your jaw, clenching your teeth. Count to five, release and repeat once more. Become aware of all your face and any difference you feel. Raise your shoulders to your ears, tensing the muscles of your shoulders and neck. Release and relax the muscles. Notice any difference and repeat once more. Raise your left hand and elbow off the floor/bed. Make a fist and increase the tension in your hand, forearm, upper arm. Count to five and let go, allowing the hand to fall back on the floor/ bed. Notice any difference between your left and right hand and repeat once more. Repeat the same with the right hand and arm. Now contract the muscles of the chest – notice the effect it has on your breathing. Relax. Flatten and tighten the muscles of your stomach – count to five – relax and exhale. Lift your left foot and leg off the floor by about six inches. Push your foot away from you, tensing the muscles of the foot, leg and thigh. Count to five. Let go and allow the leg to drop down on the floor. Repeat once more on the left side, then again, twice on the right.

In addition to tensing and releasing, this exercise can be repeated and a stretching element introduced into the exercises. Following this exercise, you can begin to guide yourself into a deeper state of muscular relaxation as follows:

Exercise III
Starting with your forehead and face, let go of any tension, relax the muscles of the face – relax the muscles of the jaw. Check that your teeth are not too tightly clenched together. Allow the tongue to lie away from the roof of the mouth. Allow your head and shoulders to fall back easily on the floor. Relax the upper arms, lower arms, hands and fingers. Let go of any tension in your chest and abdomen. Allow your breathing to become diaphragmatic. Breathe smoothly, regularly, rhythmically and without effort. – *Pause* – Relax the muscles of your feet, legs and thighs and allow your whole body to be supported by the floor and bring the focus of your attention to your breathing. – *Pause* – If any thoughts, worries or concerns come into your mind, allow them to come; then allow them to go, bringing your attention back to your breathing. – *Pause* – When you are ready to finish, bring some feeling back into your fingers and toes – take a few deeper breaths in. Open your eyes gently and sit up slowly and gradually.

This series of exercises should form the basis for many of the subsequent exercises in this book. They are a way of helping the body return to a more relaxed and healthy state. Muscles and breathing affect the way we sit, stand, lie and sleep, etc., and of course, the reverse is also true. Cultivating the art of being in a relaxed posture with a regular rhythmical form of diaphragmatic breathing throughout the day and night is a habit that comes from increasing our awareness together with regular practice of these simple exercises. Below we provide a simple guide of everyday activities in which it is possible to practise a type of 'relaxation in action'.

Sitting

Choose the right sort of chair where your back and seat are well supported. Preferably your spine should be kept straight and balanced easily on your hips. It is helpful to imagine a string coming out of the top of your spine, keeping your spine vertical and suspended over your pelvis. Your legs should be able to reach the floor and if you are sitting at a desk for some time it is better to uncross your legs and if necessary place a small cushion underneath them. Sitting in an armchair or easy chair may look comfortable but often will produce tension around the shoulders and pelvic muscles as they are commonly unsupported. However you are sitting, get into the habit of checking the state of your muscles and guiding yourself into a relaxed posture using your breathing. If your abdomen is kept tight and your shoulders and spine curved, you will find it more difficult to breathe with your diaphragm. Some people find sitting on the floor the most comfortable way of sitting and it is worth experimenting. Raising your pelvis with a small cushion will help in this position as well.

Reading and writing

We each have our favourite positions for these activities, but long periods of concentrating may cause you to tense your face or clench your jaw. Writing with your hand relaxed and not gripping the pen or pencil is not difficult once you bring your awareness to the muscles involved. Take a few moments to ensure you are breathing regularly and have not stopped at some point in the book.

Watching television

This is one of the most frequent activities, especially for children. If you do watch television a lot, make sure you have a chair that supports you well. The light in the room should be sufficient for you not to need to tighten your facial muscles or screw up your eyes. If you have difficulty in seeing, then have your eyesight checked. Falling asleep in front of the television may give the impression of being relaxed, but it often leads to cramped tense muscles, vague low-grade headaches and difficulty in sleeping in a bed. Learning to choose which programme you want to watch and switching the television off before the national anthem is a way of taking responsibility for yourself directly. The content of the television programmes has been blamed for the increase in violence and disturbed behaviour present in our society. Whilst there may be some truth in this claim, it is equally true that the passivity involved in the act of watching television can be equally harmful.

Driving

The car is a feature of modern life and the sort of car we own, how we look after it and drive it reflects in some way our personality. Watching a person drive, how they sit, grip the steering wheel, the expression they have on their face, will give you a great deal of information as to how relaxed or stressed they are. Some car seats seem to have been designed especially to produce low back pain and muscle tension. Next time you drive your car, take a few moments to become aware of how you are sitting and whether your face is tense or relaxed. Some of the earliest research done on stress was a study of car drivers and bus drivers. It demonstrated how high levels of noradrenaline, the stress hormone, were present in the blood during these activities. Waiting in a traffic jam is an excellent opportunity for practising diaphragmatic breathing. On long car journeys with children, reducing the level of stress may be the most important factor in determining the success of the holiday or trip. Opening the window to increase ventilation, singing or playing a quiz game may all help to relieve boredom as well as to exercise the muscles. Practising a head roll exercise (described in the next chapter – page 66) is helpful in decreasing the tension in the back of the neck. Most important, however, is the check you keep on your breathing – remember it is the most important thing of the holistic response.

Standing and waiting

These are activities which we each of us no doubt have to do quite frequently. Check and see that your weight is distributed evenly, that your move from one foot to the other every now and again. Shoes are obviously important in this context. For women it may be necessary to think seriously about avoiding stiletto heels when there is going to be a lot of standing about. Fortunately fashion is beginning to take health into account and there are a number of sensible, attractive shoes for women in the shops now. Help your body by choosing clothes and shoes that will not cramp your muscles or stop you breathing easily. If you develop any tension or cramp in the muscles, learn how to relieve the distress by consciously relaxing that part. It can help to imagine you are breathing into the part of the body that is tense or painful and that as you breathe out you allow the part to relax. This technique is also useful for helping you reduce the pain involved in a headache or sore tooth or minor injury. A certain amount of the pain is related to the tenseness of the muscles. Reducing the tenseness will help to reduce the pain.

Answering the telephone

For some this can be a very tense-making activity. The interruption it can cause can be enormous. Not being able to see the other person reduces the directness of communication possible. Learning to count to three or taking a good breath in and out before answering the phone can help. Checking your breathing whilst talking is important – sometimes you will find your face or hands have tensed up. Learning to say *no* or asking the person to ring back if you are occupied with another activity may be an appropriate method of protecting yourself from an unwanted stressor. Choosing not to answer the telephone when you are at home during the weekend or devoting yourself to your family is also a habit worth cultivating.

Washing up

This is a chore that causes many a 'tense state' in families, yet if it is approached with the right attitude and carried out slowly with care, in a relaxed state and with regular breathing, it can become quite a pleasure. The warm water helps to relax the body – try it and see.

Brushing teeth, washing face, taking showers and bathing

These are all activities we engage in daily or weekly. They provide an excellent opportunity for increasing awareness of our bodies, practising relaxation in action and decreasing muscle tension. Next time you brush your teeth, take a moment to observe what you are doing – how fast or slow do you brush your teeth, is your face tense or relaxed as you are involved in this activity? Slow the whole process down – or even better, brush your teeth with the other hand and notice the difference. As you wash your face, learn to use your fingers to check the tension of your muscles. Begin to massage your face gently, especially over the forehead and eyes. The use of massage as a way of both learning about your body and looking after it will be described in some detail in another chapter. Taking a shower or having a bath may be dictated by which you prefer and why. Lying in a warm bath is indeed very relaxing, but having a shower can help to invigorate and raise your energy in a way that a hot bath does not. In both, the conscious process of relaxing the muscles and breathing with the diaphragm will increase the benefits derived.

Going to the lavatory

It is surprising how such a universal habit practised by everyone at least once or twice a day is so rarely discussed. Yet the habits and posture we adopt can have an enormous impact on our health. It is difficult to discuss this area of our daily life without discussing diet but, for the moment, let us agree to include it in our discussion from the point of view of muscles, posture, tension. No doubt the way we were brought up and potty-trained play a large part in the way we carry out these activities. Do we sit upright on the toilet seat, do we lean forward and strain, do we hold our breath or not? Having an upright toilet, a recent addition to our life-style, may have made the act of defecation more 'civilised', but it has been responsible for a number of negative consequences. Defecation whilst sitting as opposed to squatting requires more pressure to be exerted. The rectum is at a different angle in these two postures and the change in position together with a reduction in the fibre content of our diet is thought to be responsible for such conditions as piles, varicose veins, hiatus hernia, gall stones – all diseases of western civilisations, not found in so-called 'primitive' communities. We pay a high price for our so-called civilised acts of defecation. No one is likely to introduce a 'continental-style' toilet into their homes, so we have to continue with our present state but keep in mind the problems they can create.

Lying down, resting, sleeping

Lying down is not necessarily resting, resting is not necessarily relaxing, and sleeping is not necessarily restful. If we are to benefit from all these activities, then we need to approach them with a little more understanding than we normally do. Again the important elements are awareness and breathing. The actual bed we sleep or lie on is also important – a firm well-supported mattress that does not sag in the middle, the appropriate number of pillows. We will spend a third of our lifetime in bed sleeping, so it is worthwhile paying some attention to this activity.

Sleep

Sleep disorders are probably the most common problem known to man. At present in the UK it is calculated that in one night in seven sleep is aided through a sleeping tablet or tranquilliser. In Scotland over 50% of women over 65 take a sleeping tablet of some kind. Over a third of children when questioned reported difficulty in sleeping or distressful dreams and nightmares. From between 7 to 10 million people in Britain experience difficulty with sleeping fairly often.

What is sleep?

Not all animals sleep, but all humans do to a varying degree. Depriving humans of sleep can produce no ill-effects for quite a while and some individuals regularly need only 2–3 hours sleep a night. It is safe to say that during sleep the body has an opportunity to rest and the mind has an opportunity to refrain from conscious activity. Notice, we use the word opportunity because for some people, sleep is neither physically nor mentally restful. Our theories about sleep have been revolutionised in the last thirty or so years with the development of the EEG (electro-encephalogram) and the use of film cameras in sleep laboratories.

Sleep cycle

The EEG is an instrument that can measure electrical activity from the brain during sleep. Using this instrument it has been possible to discover that during sleep certain phases or stages occur. Each stage is characterised by a certain type of electrical activity, and the stage of sleep in which we dream has been called the REM stage (because it is accompanied by rapid eye movements). Thus we now know that every person dreams even though they may not remember their dreams. Certain drugs including sleeping tablets can cause a disturbance in the REM type sleep which can have repercussions for the rest of the sleep cycle.

The first phase of sleep is characterised by the presence of alpha waves on the EEG and is associated with drowsiness and light sleep. Over a period of 30–60 minutes the electrical activity changes to include what are known as 'sleep spindles' (stages 2 and 3) and finally to stage 4 in which the electrical activity contains 'theta' waves. These cycles from 1–4 are repeated throughout the night and usually number 6–8 a night. Following stage 4, or deep sleep, there is a period lasting 10–15 minutes of REM. If people are woken up during REM sleep, other body movement may occur, changing posture in bed, turning over and on occasions penile erection. The percentage of time we spend in different phases of sleep varies with age, culture and activities undertaken during the day. How long we sleep also varies and it is difficult to answer the question 'How much sleep do I need?' directly. Nevertheless, some general guidelines can be given and the table gives the average. Often people get quite concerned that they are not sleeping enough, especially elderly people. This may be because of a number of reasons we shall explore later, but it is important to appreciate that as we get older there is a natural decline in the amount of sleep, both deep sleep and REM.

From the following tables it can be seen that as we grow older we sleep less, take more time in getting off to sleep and wake up more often during the night. Is this normal? We can only answer this question if we put sleep in the context of the whole 24 hours of our activities. Does the sleep we get allow us to perform adequately during our waking time? If we are ill or under stress, we may need more sleep to recover than those occasions when we are more relaxed. During sleep, many of our bodily processes slow down. However, during deep muscular relaxation or in meditation, the body processes are slowed down even more than during deep sleep. One of the results of practising a deep relaxation exercise before you sleep is that you may find you need less sleep than before.

Table I

Age	Average total sleep time	Average time taken to get to sleep	Average no. of wakenings per night
3– 6	9.89	14.3	Less than 1
6– 9	9.68	12.24	More than 1
10–12	9.33	17.39	Less than 1
13–15	8.08	15.78	More than 2
16–19	7.53	17.75	More than 2
20–29	7.08	17.73	More than 2
30–39	7.06	7.80	More than 1
40–49	6.79	8.91	More than 3
50–59	6.84	11.06	More than 5
60–69	6.77	12.38	More than 5
70–79	6.55	23.0	More than 7

Why is sleep disturbed?

Table II lists the types of sleep disturbances that have been described and most of us will have experienced several of them. Snoring and sleep apnoea are two conditions recently discovered to be associated with clinical complications. Snoring occurs because the sleeper for some reason begins to breathe through his mouth and causes a disturbance in the air-flow at the back of his throat. Sleep apnoea is the name given to the occasions when the sleeper stops breathing altogether. This may last for anything up to 90 seconds. But these conditions are associated with chest breathing and a higher incidence of heart complications, sudden death and strokes. A study on an intensive-care ward in hospitals showed that almost all coronary patients were chest breathers, a higher proportion of them snored and those that snored had periods of sleep apnoea, a higher proportion had heart irregularities which included total stopping of the heart. One sleep disorder that is not often recognised as one is oversleeping or hypersomnia, associated with deficiency in waking and low energy during the day.

Table II

Types of sleep disturbance
Difficulty getting off to sleep
Waking up during sleep

Waking up tired
Over-sleeping (hypersomnia)
Disturbed dreams and nightmares
Sleep talking and sleep walking
Snoring
Sleep apnoea
Bed wetting

Table III lists some of the causes of sleep disturbances and before you can begin to help yourself with your own sleeping pattern, it is important to identify precisely what sort of sleep disturbance you have and attempt to understand why it is occurring.

Table III

Causes of sleep disturbance

Illness

Change in climate	{ temperature storms etc.
Change in environment	{ noise new bed
Food and drink	{ overeating alcohol liquids stimulant food

Life situations
Loss or bereavement
Marital difficulties
Mental overactivity
Depressive illness
Unresolved conflicts
Going to bed tense
Sexual frustration

Improving your sleep
Invariably most people start to worry about their sleep when they are having difficulties and it is often the worst time to start.

Difficulty in sleeping can usually be traced to some problem during the day. Remember that part of the holistic approach is about recognising the interconnection between parts – day and night.

Start by identifying the cause of your sleep difficulty. Have you overeaten, is the room too hot, is the bed uncomfortable, are you worried about something in the past or the future, is your wife/husband snoring or restless and keeping you awake? Some couples find that sleeping in separate beds improves their sleep pattern and there is no law that states that married couples should sleep in a double bed. Is your sleep disturbance temporary and due to some recent change, or do you have a long-standing problem that may require professional help?

(1) Things to do during the night before going to sleep
– listen to a favourite piece of music
– avoid stimulant drinks before sleep – coffee, tea, cocoa
– avoid too many liquids, especially if bladder capacity is low
– practise a breathing and relaxation routine (exercise)
– practise a tension-releasing routine
– go for a brisk walk
– avoid starting an argument or important discussion
– write down any immediate worries or anxieties on a piece of paper
– read a book that is gripping
– do not panic

(2) Things to do if you wake up
– get up and go to the toilet
– practise a breathing routine
– write down any thoughts or worries on a piece of paper
– choose a mental image – your last holiday, a favourite film, a pleasing scene, and focus your mind on the details
– if this is frequent, have a cassette tape recorder by you and play a relaxing piece of music or relaxation tape with earphones
– if you are very tense, get up and expel some of the energy through some form of physical activity

(3) Things to do during the day time
– recognise you have a difficulty and decide to deal with it during the day as well as at night

– check your exercise routine (see Chapter 4)
– check your diet (see Chapter 5)
– examine the reasons why you may not be sleeping
    – unresolved psychological problem
    – marital conflict
    – loss of a loved one
– be honest with yourself but also be kind
– seek the help of a doctor, counsellor, friend, psychologist

(4) Aids to sleeping

Hot drinks Hot milk is said to be helpful and should be tried, as should the other drinks such as Ovaltine or Horlicks. Herbal remedies for insomnia include honey, cinnamon, rose-hip, camomile, etc.

Tranquillisers, sleeping tablets This is a vast subject and we do not intend to give specific details of the drugs that are available. There is no doubt that too many of these substances are prescribed but also that many of them are never used. The occasional use of a mild tranquilliser or non-addictive sleeping tablet is perfectly appropriate and reasonable. In times of emotional crisis through divorce or bereavement it may be difficult to avoid their use and if you can accept that part of being human involves a certain amount of suffering which is not abnormal, so much the better. You are likely to come out of that experience stronger and more able to help your fellow human beings. The lack of close emotional support may make this more difficult and recourse to drugs may be a second best. Make sure you receive the help of a doctor, counsellor or psychologist if you find yourself requiring regular sleeping medication.

4

EXERCISE – A HOLISTIC APPROACH

There has been a gradual increase in our involvement in sport and exercise. 'Sport for All' is becoming more than just a slogan, and the increase in leisure centres and sports clubs is an indication of how extensive this change in our attitudes has become. Some people, however, when they think of exercising, think of effort, sweat, hearty jolly laughter and boredom. Although most of us know that regular exercise is an important ingredient of a healthy life, some people are still reluctant to give time to this pursuit and the nearest they get to exercise is watching other people perform either on the television or in a sports ground. Watching an expert in sport, be it football, athletics or yoga, can also serve to put them off the whole idea of trying it for themselves. The expert's perfect performance may only help to make them feel more inefficient and inadequate and prevent them from experimenting.

The first and probably most important aspect of any form of exercise you do is that you should enjoy it. The second important factor is that you should do it with some *awareness*. We have seen how jogging, which was hailed as an activity for everyone where body-mind-spirit came together in an effortless pursuit of wholeness, has been turned into a commercial enterprise of multicoloured track suits, rigid training schedules and marathons. The *joy* and *awareness* of the exercise has been replaced by competitions, time-barriers, shoulds and musts. A holistic approach to exercise is more about increasing our awareness of our body, its strengths as well as its limitations. To that extent it is more important how we exercise rather than whether we exercise at all. The individual who becomes a 'weekend warrior' can find that he causes himself more harm than good. Arriving home on Friday having taken no exercise at all during the week, and then running or playing squash for a long time over the weekend, is not the best way of 'keeping fit'. As I hope we shall be able to show, it is possible for everyone, however old or however unfit or infirm, to be able to introduce some form of exercise or physical awareness into their weekly routine. Before we do that, let us look at some of the specific benefits and problems involved with exercise.

Effect on heart and lungs

Regular exercising which involves increasing the respiration and pulse rate will, over a period of time, have an effect on the *resting-pulse-rate*, *blood pressure*, *heart muscle tone* and *efficiency of the lungs*. In addition, regular exercise can increase the number and size of blood vessels to the muscles, reduces cholesterol and increases the total amount of blood available to the different tissues of the body.

Resting-pulse-rate

This is a measure of the number of times your heart pumps in one minute whilst you are in a resting state. It varies with age, sex and fitness level. It can be easily calculated by placing two fingers (middle and index) over the 'radial artery' which can be found just above the wrist joint on the base of the thumb. Count the number of beats for 10 seconds, then multiply by six. You now have your resting-pulse-rate per minute.

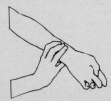

If you find your resting pulse-rate to be over 100 you should consult your doctor. In addition, your resting-pulse-rate will give you a guide as to how careful you must be in taking up a vigorous form of exercise. At this point, it might be helpful to add that it is better to have 5–10 minutes exercise routine 3–4 times a week than one hour at the weekend.

Blood pressure

Amongst other things, your blood pressure is an indication of the 'tone' of your blood vessels and helps to determine with what force your heart has to pump in order to enable the blood to circulate round your body. Generally it is not possible to take your own blood pressure, although there are some home instruments on the market. Blood pressure is measured by squeezing a cuff over the upper arm and either feeling the pulse or listening with a stethoscope over the artery for the blood to flow again once the cuff is released. The blood pressure measurement includes two figures: the systolic figure is the first measurement and reflects the age and state of the wall of the artery. As we grow older, the arteries stiffen and the systolic blood pressure rises a little. This is normal and generally speaking an acceptable figure is 100 + your age. The systolic measurement increases with anxiety and exercise. The diastolic figure is the lower figure and reflects the tension in the small muscles surrounding the medium-sized arteries. This figure should generally be below 90, although like the systolic figure it tends to rise with age. Most doctors will consider treating your blood pressure with drugs if the systolic pressure is over 170 (lower if you are 60 or younger) and the diastolic is above 100. However, there are many other ways of reducing high blood pressure and regular exercise is one of them.

Heart as   Organ
pump   (muscle)

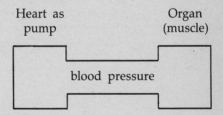

blood pressure

Lung efficiency

The lungs are the organs where oxygen is taken up by the blood and carbon dioxide is removed and expelled. The exchange of oxygen is made more efficient when the breathing is regular, rhythmical and full. 'Being fit' results in being able to take deeper breaths and aerating more lung tissue each time. In the previous chapter we mentioned the importance of *diaphragmatic breathing* in relaxation and stress control. Being aware of the breath during exercise is equally important and can enhance the beneficial effects to a great degree. Little guidance is given on how we should breathe during exercise and it is important to emphasise that in all but the most strenuous forms of exercise it is helpful to maintain the regular rhythmical form of diaphragmatic breathing. One very good precaution is to exercise only to the extent that if you had to stop, you could continue a conversation without being short of breath (the talk test). You do not have to tire yourself out or pant to benefit from exercise and more damage is done by overdoing the exercise than by maintaining an easy, relaxed approach to whatever exercise you are engaged in.

Heart muscle tone

There has been much work done recently in the use of exercise following heart attacks. Heart attacks (coronary thrombosis, myocardial infarction) are the result of a small clot or thrombosis blocking the blood supply to a portion of heart muscle. The heart muscle dies and causes the pain associated with heart attacks. Angina is the condition when the heart muscle is deprived of sufficient oxygen but does not actually die – like 'cramp' in any muscle. If a large part of the heart muscle dies, then the heart can lose its efficiency and the condition known as 'heart failure' occurs. Supervised exercise programmes following heart attacks help to restore the efficiency of the heart by increasing the muscle tone and increasing the size of blood vessels taking oxygen to the heart muscle. If you have had heart problems, then it is important to seek guidance before embarking on a fitness programme. You do not have to wait for your first heart attack to do the same thing! Men who regularly exercise have a lower incidence of heart attacks than men who do not.

Effect on muscles, tendons, ligaments and bones

One can understand the effect exercise has on these parts of the body if one remembers the effect of no exercise at its most extreme – lying in bed because of an illness. After a while, the muscles begin to waste away and lose their tone and strength. The tendons and ligaments shorten and tighten and the joints become less flexible and stiffer. The bones begin to lose their 'calcium' and become softer and more liable to fractures. In addition, constipation develops. Many of the problems of the elderly are the result not of 'old age' itself but of the lack of exercise and the poor advice given to them. Even so, more people injure themselves, pull a muscle or ligament, twist an ankle or knee, or break a bone as a result of poorly performed exercise than from doing no exercise, the reason being that exercise, like everything else about the holistic approach, has to be carried out with awareness: awareness not just of the precautions and safety measures one needs to take, but awareness of one's body. It is a matter of 'listening to your body', realising the important difference between the discomfort experienced from underused muscles and stretched ligaments as opposed to the pain from having stretched too far. If we get into the habit of listening to our bodies, the lessons we can learn can often be applied to our personal and emotional lives as well. The important precautionary steps to take before any form of exercise involve stretching and warming up, and they will be described on page 58.

Effects on weight, diet and cholesterol

One of the reasons a number of people take up exercise is to lose weight. Unfortunately, the arithmetic of calories has been used to discourage people. You have to run nearly two miles to lose 200 calories (3 slices of bread). Stated in those terms, it is no wonder that exercise routines are not popular amongst the overweight. If you are overweight and want to lose it, then a good diet is obviously important. It is true nevertheless that a diet with an exercise programme is particularly helpful, not only because of the reduction in calories required but because exercise actually helps to control appetite.

Cholesterol is a fatty substance normally circulating in the blood. If your diet is high in fat (dairy products – eggs, meat), then your cholesterol may be elevated. Having an elevated cholesterol increases the likelihood of developing coronary artery disease. Regular exercise is known to decrease the level of circulating cholesterol and for many people this can be the best method of restoring the levels to normality.

Effects on mood, alertness and stress

Let us simplify the use of the word 'stress' for a moment. There are times when we feel in a low mood, have little energy, feel unhappy or depressed, and then there are times when we feel tense, irritable, unable to settle or relax. Can exercise help in such situations? Let us simplify things even further and say there are times when we are in a *low energy* state and times when we are in a *high energy* state. Exercise can be used both to increase low energy states and decrease high energy states. Exercise can be used as a 'first aid' for bringing about a more balanced mood and regular exercise has been shown to improve long-standing depression as well as long-standing chronic anxiety states. Some of the benefits occur because exercise reduces the level of lactic acid (a measure of how tense we are) and increases the level of endorphins (the body's own happy pill). Releasing tension by shouting, banging, laughing or crying can be very important aids in helping to restore our equilibrium, and our culture, which emphasises 'not showing our emotions', 'keeping a stiff upper lip', can be harmful to this process. Crying is an important form of exercise whose effect is particularly helpful. Crying and sobbing change the pattern of breathing and help to relieve muscular tension. The shedding of tears helps to decrease the level of stress hormone circulating in the blood (the hormone is actually excreted in the tears).

As we shall see later on, regular breathing exercises practised at home can be a perfectly adequate form of exercise for many people unable to take up more active forms. The long-term psychological benefits of exercise occur when exercise is practised with awareness of the links between bodily states and mental states. Becoming more sensitive about the flexibility of your joints or the strength of your muscles helps to develop similar sensitivity to those psychological attributes. Learning how to stretch your body and understanding the limits of your capacities are translated to your everyday pursuits if you adopt an attitude of *awareness*. Practising exercises to balance the left and right side of your body increases your capacity to balance the different aspects of your life.

What sort of exercise?

The exercise routine you choose will be influenced by your age, general level of health, interest and past experience. Some prefer to exercise on their own, others enjoy a team sport or learning together in a class. The intensity of exercise is measured by using the unit called MET (metabolic unit). One MET is the amount of energy expended at rest which for average size men and women is about 1–1.25 calories per minute at rest. Looking at the tables below, you can work out some of the common activities you perform at home and their MET levels. A useful way of deciding on the choice of exercise is to use the scheme below:

Met Levels

OCCUPATIONAL	1	2	3	4	5	6	7	8	9	10	11
Clerical	□										
Bench assembly		□									
Truck driving			□								
Welding			□								
Production line assembly			□								
Bricklaying				□							
Carpentry				□							
Lawn mowing					□						
Digging							□				
Wood chopping								□			
Stair climbing (15 m min. carrying 10 kg)											□

Met Levels

DOMESTIC SELF-CARE	1	2	3	4	5	6	7	8	9	10	11
Machine sewing	□										
Showering, dressing		□									
Ironing		□									
Walking 3 km/hr		□									
Sweeping		□									
Walking 5 km/hr			□								
Bed making			□								
Hanging clothes			□								
Vacuuming			□								
Scrubbing floors				□							

Met Levels

SPORT	1	2	3	4	5	6	7	8	9	10	11	12	13	14	15
Billiards															
Lawn bowls															
Fishing															
Ten pin bowling															
Archery															
Golf															
Volley ball															
Cricket															
Horse riding															
Sailing															
Table tennis															
Dancing															
Badminton															
Tennis (doubles)															
Tennis (singles)															
Water skiing															
Ice/roller skating															
Scuba diving															
Swimming															
Cycling															
Rowing															
Fencing															
Gymnastics															
Football															
Basketball															
Boxing															
Judo															
Skipping 60–80/ min.															
Skipping 120–140/ min.															
Squash															

	1	2	3	4	5	6	7	8	9	10	11	12	13	14
Walking, jogging, running		4	5			6		8		10		12		km/h
One kilometre in minutes		15	12			10		7.30		6		5		4.15 mins

(1) Very intensive

These forms of exercise are usually team or competitive sports.
They provide opportunities for very active but intermittent bouts

56

of exercise. The pulse rate is variable during the exercise period and usually the emphasis is on winning the game or achieving mastery over the other team. The competitive element is emphasised and the enjoyment follows the 'result' (win or lose) rather than the exercise itself. However, the recent success of such books as *Inner Tennis* suggests that recreational sport of this kind does not always have to emphasise the competitive element.

(2) Moderate/rhythmical

In these forms of exercise there is usually a sustained, continuous, rhythmical exercise, such as swimming, running, walking, cycling, vigorous gymnastics. The pulse rate and breathing are increased and are maintained at a regular rate for a greater length of time than in the previous form. Although these forms of exercise can be competitive, by their very nature they are more likely to be pursued individually and the focus of attention is more easily maintained on the experience than on the goal. Nevertheless, as mentioned earlier, time schedules and marathons all help to diminish the joy of running or cycling for its own sake. These last two forms of exercise are generally 'aerobic', which means that your respiration and pulse rate increase during exercise. 'Aerobics', as popularised by Jane Fonda, is a special form of gymnastics and dance carried out sufficiently fast for you to need to increase your respiration. Much of the criticism levelled at aerobics has to do with the inadequacy of the warming up time and the speed at which the exercises are performed. Looking good may make you feel good, but feeling good does not require you to look like Jane Fonda or Raquel Welch.

(3) 'Static'

These forms of exercise are less intensive in the sense that they are usually non-aerobic or anaerobic. They include yoga, gymnastics, Canadian Air Force exercises, tai-chi, weight-lifting. There is little increase in respiration or pulse rate. However, they can be fairly intensive in terms of the stretching of the muscles, and anyone who has held a particular yoga posture for a long time would attest to their intensity. These exercises are usually carried out in a class or gym, but their major advantage is that they can also be carried out at home, require no special clothing and are inexpensive, if not free. By far the most popular form of exercise is yoga, which may vary from simple stretching exercises to complex postures.

(4) Breathing exercises

Finally, for those who are infirm or unfit, or who do not enjoy any of the above forms, it is possible, through the practice of a variety of breathing exercises, to maintain a level of awareness which is perfectly acceptable. These exercises will be described below.

Getting ready

This will depend somewhat on the intensity of the exercise to be undertaken and your present level of fitness. Some common-sense precautions are applicable generally: the need for comfortable clothes and the right sort of footwear; the importance of avoiding strenuous exercise including stretches after meals. Preparing mind, body and breath for exercise involves a few minutes 'warming up'.

Mental preparation

It may sound ridiculous at first, but asking yourself why you want to exercise is the first preparation required. Is it because you feel you ought to? Or because you want to keep fit? Sometimes you may make a conscious decision to exercise because you feel stressed and tense or on other occasions it may be for the enjoyment of the experience itself. And for some, the joy of competition and winning is the drive behind the wish to exercise. Competing and winning are perfectly appropriate human activities. The problem arises when the need to compete and win interfere with the enjoyment or the stress-releasing aspects of exercise. That is why *awareness* is so central to the process. It adds the dimension which allows you to participate fully in the activity and not just as a passenger or observer. To (mis)quote Lawrence Durrell, 'to realise the importance of *exercise* and get contemplative enough to enjoy it is something achieved'. So if you are running for the pleasure and experience, then leave your watch behind.

Breath preparation

Breathing helps to link body and mind. Both before and during exercise it is helpful to breathe rhythmically through the nose and with the diaphragm, especially in the repetitive and moderately intensive forms of exercise. In the very active forms of exercise it will be necessary to use both types of breathing (chest and diaphragm), but allowing the breathing to become more balanced between the periods of high intensity preserves energy and helps concentration.

Body preparation
A warm-up period of five minutes stretching before the more intensive forms of exercise (1 and 2) is necessary to prevent injury, prepare the body and improve performance.

Choosing an exercise programme
Enough has been said about the importance of enjoyment and awareness in exercise for there to be no doubt that the form of exercise must be your own choice. Most people will find amongst the four groups of exercises one form that suits them. Some will find that they enjoy and possibly need different types of exercise to meet their different needs, such as squash or tennis for a competitive, active, intense focus, and yoga or jogging for a more relaxed, balanced and pleasurable focus. It is important, before you start, to be aware of any factors which might limit your choice of exercises. These include:

General level of fitness (see below).
Presence of specific disease, e.g. heart problem.
Past injury to bones, muscles or ligaments.

In America it has been the custom to seek medical opinion before starting on an exercise programme. Whereas on occasions this is advisable, it does tend to diminish the responsibility of the individual himself for determining his own limits. Relying on the 'expert' to tell you how fit you are avoids the necessity for you to become aware of this for yourself.

Q.   TEST 1
What is your resting pulse rate?
Your resting pulse is a simple and accurate gauge of cardiovascular fitness. As your fitness level increases, your resting pulse rate will become slower, stronger and more regular. Take your pulse when you wake up in the morning, because any form of emotional or physical exertion will affect it during the day. Individual rates vary but, as a general rule, women have a slightly higher pulse

rate than men. If you find your resting pulse is over 100 beats a minute, consult your doctor immediately.

Take your pulse at your wrist (at the base of your thumb) or by feeling the artery in your neck, which is located below the ear and toward the jawbone.

A. *Resting pulse rate*

Age	20–29	30–39	40–49	50+

Men

	20–29	30–39	40–49	50+
Excellent	59 or less	63 or less	65 or less	67 or less
Good	60–69	64–71	66–73	68–75
Fair	70–85	72–85	74–89	76–89
Poor	86+	86+	90+	90+

Women

	20–29	30–39	40–49	50+
Excellent	71 or less	71 or less	73 or less	75 or less
Good	72–77	72–79	75–79	77–83
Fair	78–95	80–97	80–98	84–102
Poor	96+	98+	99+	103+

Q. TEST 2

What is your heart recovery time?

Try this simple step test to assess your aerobic fitness and stamina. The test reveals how efficiently your heart and lungs feed oxygen to your body by measuring the time it takes to slow down after it has speeded up for exercise. If your resting pulse rate is over 100 beats a minute, do not attempt this test. Step on to a stair about 20 cm (8 in.) high, then step down again, moving one foot after the other. Repeat 24 times a minute for 3 minutes. Stop and take your pulse. After resting 30 seconds, take your pulse again and consult the chart. Repeat this test after a few weeks of participation in an aerobic exercise programme and see if your heart recovers more quickly. The heart's natural capacity declines with age, so beware of exceeding the safe limits as you grow older. If at any moment you feel dizzy, nauseated or painfully breathless, stop immediately.

A. *Recovery pulse rate at 30 seconds*

Age	20–29	30–39	40–49	50+

Men

	20–29	30–39	40–49	50+
Excellent	74	78	80	83
Good	76–84	80–86	82–88	84–90
Fair	86–100	88–100	90–104	92–104
Poor	102+	102+	106+	106+

Women

	20–29	30–39	40–49	50+
Excellent	86	86	88	90
Good	88–92	88–94	80–94	92–98
Fair	99–110	95–112	96–114	100–116
Poor	112+	114+	114+	118+

Q. *TEST 3*

What is your safe maximum pulse rate?

During exercise, be sure not to exceed the following values:

Age	20–29	30–39	40–49	50+
Men	170	160	150	140
Women	170	160	150	140

Q. TEST 4

How active are you?

How often do you take physical exercise (including keep fit classes and sport) that makes you out of breath?

a. Four times or more a week
b. Two to three times a week
c. Once a week
d. Less than once a week

How far do you walk each day?

a. More than 5 km (3 miles)
b. Up to 5 km (3 miles)
c. Less than 1.6 km (1 mile)
d. Less than 0.8 km (½ mile)

How do you travel to work, the shops?

a. All the way by foot/cycle
b. Part of the way by foot/cycle
c. Occasionally by foot/cycle
d. All the way by public transport or car

When there is a choice do you?

a. Take the stairs – up and down – always
b. Take the stairs unless you have something to carry
c. Occasionally take the stairs
d. Take the lift/escalator unless it is broken

At weekends do you?

a. Spend several hours gardening/decorating/DIY/doing some sport

b. Usually only sit down for meals and in the evening
c. Take a few short walks
d. Spend most of the time sitting reading/watching TV
Do you think nothing of?
a. Doing the household chores after a day's work
b. Rushing out to the shops again if you have forgotten something
c. Getting other people to run your errands even if you have time
d. Paying for a telephone call when you could make a personal visit

---

A. *Add up your score, allowing*
4 points for every *a* answer
3 points for every *b* answer
2 points for every *c* answer
1 point for every *d* answer

20+
You are naturally very active and probably quite fit.
15–20
You are active and have a healthy attitude toward fitness.
10–15
You are only mildly active and would benefit from some more exercise.
Under 10
You are rather lazy and need to rethink your attitude toward activity. Try to reorganise your day to allow for some exercise.

Q. TEST 5
What can you do?
How long does it take you to:
1. Walk 5 km (3 miles) on level ground
   a. 1 hr 15 min (or more)

     b. 50 min to 1 hr 10 min
     c. 45 min (or less)
  2. Swim 1,000 m (1,000 yds)
     a. 50 min (or more)
     b. 40 min
     c. 20 min (or less)
  3. Run 1.6 km (1 mile) on level ground
     a. 15 min (or more)
     b. 9–14 min
     c. 8 min (or less)

A. *Scores*
  a. If you have covered the distance, you have made a start. Now keep it up until the test feels easy.
  b. You are moderately fit. If you want to improve, increase the distance and speed up gradually.
  c. You have reached a good level of fitness and are ready to start a more vigorous fitness programme.

Exercise and women

One of the many benefits of the women's movement has been the freedom it has given women to take up and compete in sports once thought to be exclusively for men. Women have been liberated from seeing their bodies solely as objects for men's pleasure and begun to enjoy yoga, gymnastics, jogging and football for themselves. There are specific issues relating to women's exercising that affect menstruation and pregnancy.

Menstruation

Many of the top women athletes find that their periods diminish and at times disappear during extensive bouts of physical activity. There is no evidence that this affects long-term fertility and periods return to normal once the exercise routine is less intensive. Period pains and premenstrual tension may well be helped by regular exercising, but the lethargy and tiredness associated with PMT may be sufficient to prevent exercising.

Pregnancy

Whilst it is important to remain fit during pregnancy, it is important not to undertake too excessive a programe, especially in the first three months. Reducing the intensity of the exercise programme, going for long walks and learning the several breathing and relaxation routines appear to be a more sensible approach to exercise during pregnancy.

Exercise programmes

Body Awareness – time 15 mins

Sway

Wear comfortable loose clothing. Remove shoes and socks. Stand with your feet apart, 12–18 inches. Close your eyes and take a few moments to settle your breath. Begin to sway slowly, first to the left and then to the right, moving at the ankles. As you sway to the left, breathe in, as you sway to the right, breathe out. Repeat 6 times.

Allow your body to come to the centre position and pause. Now begin to sway backwards and forwards. As you sway backwards, breathe in. As you sway forwards, breathe out. Repeat 6 times, then allow your body to come to the central position and pause.

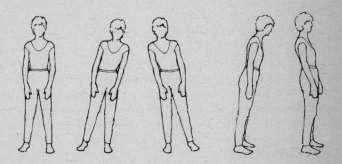

Eye rolls

Open your eyes. Focus your eyes on the top right hand corner of the room and then slowly rotate them through 360° (clockwise) keeping your head straight. Repeat 3 times. Close your eyes and observe any sensations around them. Repeat again, rotating your eyes in an anticlockwise manner. Close your eyes. Pause.

Head rolls

Let your head fall down to your chest with your chin tucked in. Slowly rotate your head to the left, bringing your ear as close to your left shoulder as you can. Take your head back and round over the right shoulder and finally bring your chin round to the front. Repeat 3 times – with your eyes closed – breathing in as you take your head back and breathing out as you bring your head forward. Repeat in the opposite direction 3 times.

Shoulder circles

Raise your arms sideways parallel to the floor. With your fingers outstretched, begin to make small circles with your fingers, rotating your arms at the shoulder joint. Gradually increase the circles, then decrease them. Repeat 3 times in one direction and 3 times in another, bringing the arms to rest by your side between times.

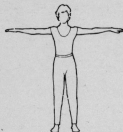

Side stretch

With your eyes closed, place your hands on the side of your legs. Bend to the left, allowing the hand to move down the leg as far as it will go. Come up slowly. Repeat 3 times, breathing out as you go down and breathing in as you come up. Repeat on the other side.

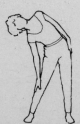

Backwards stretch

Place your hands in the small of your back supporting the back muscles. Slowly bend backwards, stretching the front muscles.

Come forward slowly. Repeat 3 times, breathing in as you bend backwards and breathing out as you bend forwards.

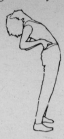

Forward stretch

Allow your hands and arms to fall forwards. Bend at the waist and allow your head to fall between your knees. Gently sway for a few moments. Breathe in – and then as you breathe out, allow the head to fall further towards the feet. Pause. Gradually come up, uncurling your back slowly.

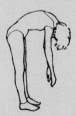

Ankle stretch

(You may need to hold on to a chair or surface for this exercise.) Lift the right leg off the floor and stretch the leg in front of you with the foot a few inches off the ground. Start rotating the ankle in one direction making small circles with your foot. Repeat 3 times in one direction, then 3 times in the other. Place the foot back on the ground and repeat on the other side.

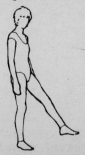

Balance
Focus your eyes on a point on the opposite side of the room.
Lift the left foot off the floor and place the foot just above the
ankle on the right leg. (You may need to hold on to a chair.)
Balance on the right leg, taking a few slow breaths in and out.
Bring the left foot back down and repeat on the other side.

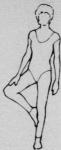

Stretching Exercises (warm up before jogging or other more vigorous exercise)

Hamstring stretch
Bend at the waist, clasping the backs of the calves with your
hands. Hold for up to 10 seconds and repeat 5 times.

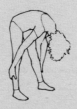

Thigh muscle stretch
Bend the left knee and stretch right leg out as far as you can
go. Balance body over left knee and hold for 3–5 seconds. Keep
right foot flat on the floor. Repeat other side.

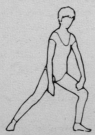

Calf stretch

Place hands against a wall standing 18″ away. Support body with your hands and gradually, with knees locked, bring your pelvis forward. Hold for a few seconds and repeat 3–5 times.

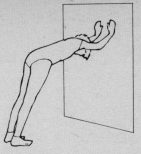

Arm circling

Lift arms to the side and make 3–5 vigorous circles with both arms. Repeat in both directions.

Breathing exercises

(1) Diaphragmatic breathing (as described in Chapter 2)

(2) Full breath (Diaphragm – Chest – clavicle)

Stand up straight with arms by your side. Begin by breathing in to the count of three with your diaphragm. Now continue to breathe in, expanding your chest to another count of three. Finally expand the upper part of your chest and lower neck again to the count of three. Breathe out, slowly reversing the process (clavicle – chest – diaphragm). Repeat 3 times.

(3) 'Bellows' breathing

This exercise should be performed with care, and if you experience any dizziness you should stop. The abdominal muscles are used to force air in and out like 'bellows'.
(1) Sit upright with head, neck and trunk in a straight line.
(2) Forcefully contract your abdominal muscles, expelling air through your nostrils.
(3) Forcefully push out the abdominal muscles and breathe in deeply and quickly.
(4) Repeat this forceful inhalation and exhalation, no more than six times to begin with.
(5) Gradually increase the number as you perfect the process.

(4) Alternate nostril breathing

This exercise helps to keep the nostrils clear and if repeated frequently will keep the body and mind in a state of balance. The breathing is diaphragmatic throughout.

(1) Sit comfortably with head, neck and trunk straight.
(2) Clear each nostril by closing first the right and then the left and exhaling moderately forcefully out of each one in turn.
(3) Close the left nostril with the left index finger.
(4) *Exhale* gently out of the right nostril.
(5) Close the right nostril with the index finger.
(6) *Inhale* through the left nostril.
(7) Close the left nostril.
(8) Exhale gently through right nostril.
(9) Repeat steps (4)–(8) three times.
(10) Inhale through right nostril.
(11) Close right nostril.
(12) Exhale through left nostril.
(13) Close left nostril.
(14) Inhale through right nostril.
(15) Repeat steps (11)–(14) three times.

There should be no pause between inhalation and exhalation. The breathing should be soundless, smooth and rhythmical.

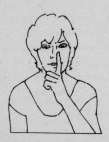

Strengthening exercises

Push-ups   (shoulder and chest muscles)
(a)   *Table*   Find a secure table or ledge.
            Stand 2 feet away and place outstretched arms on surface.
            Bend the elbows and allow the chest to come close to the surface of the table.
            Straighten the arms, pushing the body away.
            Repeat 6–10 times.

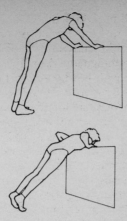

(b) *Floor* Lie face down on a carpet, mat or rug with feet stretched out behind you a few inches apart.
Place palms on floor next to the shoulders. Push yourself up, keeping your back straight and your arms straight.
Initially you may wish to keep your knees on the floor.

Sit-ups

(a) *Chair* Find a chair with a straight back and sit with head, neck and trunk straight. Place feet on the floor, keeping the knees together. Raise the knees and at the same time bring the forehead down to touch the knees or as close to them as you can manage. Bring the feet back to the floor and straighten the back. Repeat 6 times.

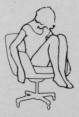

(b) *Floor* Lie on the floor on your back, feet slightly apart. Bend the left knee and bring it towards your abdomen at the same time as bringing your forehead forward.

71

Keep your hands either by your side or folded behind your head.
Bring the leg and head back to the floor.
Repeat 3 times on left and then on the right and finally 3 times with both legs at the same time.

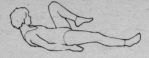

Arch-ups (back muscles)
Lie on the floor face down, hands by your side, feet together.
Gradually raise one leg off the floor from the hip keeping the leg straight.
Lower and repeat 3 times.
Repeat on the other side.
Repeat both legs together.
Repeat and at the same time lift the trunk off the floor arching the back, keeping the hands by your side.
Repeat 3 times.

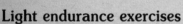

Light endurance exercises
Stair climbing/walking/jogging/running programme
Points to remember:
(1) Enjoy your exercise.
(2) Do it with awareness.
(3) Know your strengths and limitations.
(4) Warm up before you start.
(5) Cool down after you finish.
(6) Co-ordinate your mind (thoughts and feelings) and your body (movement and speed) with your breath (regular and diaphragmatic).
(7) 10 mins, three times a week is more beneficial than ½ hour at the weekend.
(8) Be creative and develop your own routine.
Stair climbing
(a) Climb stairs rather than take a lift.
(b) If you have stairs at home, spend 5 minutes a day climbing up and down. Start slowly and gradually increase the pace

and the time spent on this exercise to 15 minutes. You can make this exercise as brisk as you like, but the important factor is co-ordinating your movement awareness and breathing.

Walking

(a) Walk to the bus stop, railway station, tube or place of work. Walk to the shops and possibly arrange for any heavy shopping to be delivered. Explore the Ramblers Association or join a walking group in your area. The following exercise programme is recommended by the National Heart, Lung and Blood Institute, Bethesda, USA, but you can develop one that suits your needs.

Jogging/Walking

There is no doubt that for many adults, this activity has enhanced both their physical and mental well-being. However, it has led to many minor and, on occasion, serious health problems. If you are going to jog, jog because you want to, jog with awareness. Know your limitations, learn to enjoy the long, slow jog as well as the jog with your wife/husband/friend. You may like to join a running club and for many the participation in a 'fun run' or marathon can be a high point in their lives. Do not allow other people to ridicule your efforts but at the same time be clear as to why you are running. There are many guides, programmes, routines available. The most extensive and detailed are outlined in Ken Cooper's *Aerobics* and *Aerobics for Women*. Some of them are daunting and can put people off even starting. Remember it is much better to develop your own routine than to follow slavishly with a watch and pedometer someone else's. Experiment with walking slowly, 'race walking', slow jogging and running. Vary your course and learn about your neighbourhood. Once a week or month, give yourself a longer time and run/jog/walk a greater distance, allowing your exercise routine to become a 'meditational' exercise as well as a physical one.

5

DIET AND NUTRITION – A HOLISTIC APPROACH

Your liver has no teeth

Open any of the hundreds of books, guides and almanacs on diet and you will find detailed instructions on what you should eat and what food you should avoid. The major difficulty people face is deciding which one to follow. There appear to be as many books extolling one diet as there are telling you that the same diet is unhealthy. Each year there is a series of new discoveries informing you that what was once thought to be healthy is now thought to be harmful. Most of what is written is about the content of food, and very little on the process of eating, from buying the food to preparing it, cooking it and finally eating it. As important as the state of the food is the state the body/mind is in when the food is being eaten. This is a theme we have constantly underlined in these chapters and is well illustrated by the following example.

A few years ago a group of nutritional scientists were experimenting with a high fat diet and the development of atherosclerosis (fatty plaques in the arteries that cause heart attacks). They fed a group of rabbits a very high diet in fat and then sacrificed them to find out how far they had developed the fatty plaques and where these fatty-plaques were deposited. Some of the rabbits had developed much less atherosclerosis than others and the researchers were puzzled by this as all the rabbits had been fed the same diet. They repeated the experiment and found the same result, but observed that the group of rabbits with less atherosclerosis were fed by a different lab-technician from the ones who had developed the expected amount. At first they thought she was feeding them something different, so they repeated the experiment yet again and observed her closely. What they saw was that before she fed the rabbits this very high fat diet, she would take them out of their cages and stroke them, calming them down and reducing their fear and stress. How many of us rush our meals, whilst reading or arguing or thinking about the next appointment. We may even find we have eaten our meal without knowing what it was we have eaten. Snacking in front of the television is a common way of reducing any conscious control over the eating. Arriving home from a busy and stressful day and immediately sitting down to a meal is a common pattern for many of us. Indeed, food is a common source of comfort and diets that do not pay sufficient attention to this fact are doomed to fail. Saying grace before a meal is not very common nowadays. The few moments of silence not only provided a way of saying thank you but allowed the individuals to settle down and quieten the body processes before eating. So before we actually go into any details about the content of food, let us carry out a small experiment which will help to raise our awareness – yes, that word again – about the process of eating.

Conscious eating exercise

You can do this exercise with other members of your family, or on your own, but find a quiet room where you will be undisturbed for 10–15 minutes. Choose a fresh apple or orange and cut the fruit into wedges, putting them on a plate. Sit down in front of the plate, make yourself comfortable and close your eyes. Spend a few moments quietening your breathing and letting go of any tension in your body, especially your face and hands. Allow your breathing to become deep and rhythmical and, with your eyes still closed, pick up a piece of fruit with your fingers, become aware of the texture and edges – pause for a few moments. Then bring the piece of fruit to just below your nose and take in any smells. Try and see if you can pick out different smells from different parts of the fruit – pause for a few moments and become aware of any changes in your breathing. Now bring the fruit to your lips and tongue and explore the fruit again. Can you determine anything different? Is your tongue more sensitive than your lips? What sensations do you experience in your mouth or abdomen? Pause for a few moments. Now begin to chew a small piece of the fruit slowly and carefully. Take care to chew slowly and become aware of the tension in your jaws and face as you are chewing. When the piece of fruit is sufficiently chewed, swallow it and then pause. Allow your attention to focus on the whole process from the beginning of this exercise to the final swallow – then repeat it once more.

Now we don't have to spend that amount of time on the process of eating, but learning to settle oneself down and being careful to chew well and slowly will certainly allow one to benefit from the food being eaten. For those who are on a diet, this exercise is a particularly good method of reducing the amount of food we eat. Of all the many things wrong with our diet the two least emphasised are these – *We eat too much and we pay little attention to how we eat*. It is much easier to blame the government or the manufacturer for putting additives and preservatives in food than it is to take responsibility ourselves for the way we eat. Have you ever stopped and asked yourself 'Why do I eat?'? How many of the reasons below apply to you?

WHY DO WE EAT ?

Comfort	Social reasons
Boredom	Enjoyment
Habit	Depression
Hunger	Relieve tension
To change your mood	

Can you list other reasons?
Which are specific to you?

How has our diet changed over the last hundred years and does this change have anything to do with the problems we read so much about? If we look at Table I we can see how our current diet compares with those of our ancestors and those living in a rural community.

TABLE I

Fat 15%–20%	Fat 10%–15%	Fat 40%
Starch 50%–70%	Sugar 5% Starch 60%–70%	Sugar 20%
		Starch 25%–30%
Protein 15%–20%	Protein 15%–20%	Protein 15%–20%

Salts/d	1	5–15	15
Fibre g/d	40	60–120	20
	Hunter/gathers Pre 'civilisation'	*Peasant/agriculture communities*	*Western 'civilised' communities*

Now if we look at the patterns of eating since the Second World War, the following facts emerge:

> There has been an 80% increase in consumption of soft drinks, 70% increase in consumption of potato crisps. At the same time there has been a 25% decrease in consumption of dairy products, fruits and vegetables. We can now construct a list of guidelines to healthy eating which should serve as the basis for some of the more detailed descriptions that follow. It is important to underline that these are guidelines. Too many people become over-anxious about the food they eat and develop guilt feelings if they have a piece of chocolate or the occasional cream bun. A good guide to keeping the guidelines is, 'If you can't break the rules graciously you can't keep them graciously'.

Guidelines

Carbohydrates

Carbohydrates are the major source of 'quick energy'.

Carbohydrates are broken down in the body into one of three simple sugars (monosaccharides). These simple sugars are *glucose*, *galactose* and *fructose*. The sugar you add to your cereal

or coffee is called *sucrose* and is a combination of two monosaccharides, *glucose* and *fructose*. All carbohydrates of whatever source
are eventually broken down to glucose. Glucose is used by the
body for an immediate source of energy – it is the body's fuel
and it is stored in the liver and muscles.

TABLE II

Cereals –	Wheat	Rye
	Barley	Buckwheat
	Oats	Millett
	Corn	
Rice		
Potatoes		
Bananas		

Table II lists the sources of carbohydrates available – most are
from cereal crops – and the list includes all the starchy food we
eat from time to time. Starch is a complex carbohydrate. A
complex carbohydrate is one which is made up of a series of
simple sugars. These are arranged in an intricate pattern and
the enzymes present in the saliva, stomach and intestines have
to break the complex chains of 'sugars' down to the simple
sugars (glucose, fructose and galactose) before they can be
absorbed by the body.

TABLE III

MONOSACCHARIDES	DISACCHARIDES
Glucose	Sucrose (Glucose + Fructose)
Galactose	Lactose (Glucose + Galactose)
Fructose	Maltose (Glucose + Gluctose)

Now one of the major changes that has occurred in our diets is
that our sources of carbohydrates have altered (see Table IV).

TABLE IV

	CHO	CHO	CHO
Starch	68	49	47
Sugar	32	51	53
	1960	1969	1979

In 1960, 68% of our carbohydrates came in the form of complex starches, while in 1979 this figure was only 47%. We are eating much more of simple sugars than before. We eat on average 120 lbs of sugar a year, which works out to one teaspoon per hour day and night. Why is eating simple sugars harmful? Surely the body has to do less work in 'breaking down' the food before it is absorbed and this must help in the long run. Unfortunately the reverse is true. It appears that 10–15% of the population is sucrose sensitive. This means that if their diet is high in simple or refined sugar, their bodies respond by secreting a higher level of insulin (the hormone that deals with the sugar in the blood) than normal. If this continues for a long time, there is good evidence that they will develop diabetes. A rapid rise of blood sugar that occurs after eating a meal high in refined sugar is followed by a rapid fall in blood sugar. This can be accompanied by 'mood swings' – feeling excitable and nervous, then feeling down and depressed. The fall in blood sugar is occasionally accompanied by a lower level of blood sugar than normal (hypoglycaemia).

Some doctors now believe that it is the high sugar content of our diet that predisposes us to atherosclerosis rather than the high fat. What is definitely known is that the majority of our dental problems could be reduced if we reduced our intake of sweets and sugar. Another equally important factor is that if we do have a diet high in refined carbohydrate, many of the calories in our diet are 'empty'. What is meant by this is that many of the nutrients (vitamins, minerals) which are present in the more complex form of carbohydrates are absent, but because the diet contains sufficient and at times too many calories, our 'hunger' is satisfied but we build up a long-term deficiency in many of the necessary trace elements (zinc, cadmium, etc.). Similarly a diet high in refined carbohydrates tends to be one which is low in fibre content and this adds to the problems, as we shall describe later in the section on fibre.

Reducing the refined carbohydrate in our diets involves:

    (a) cutting down on pastries, sweets, cakes, biscuits;
    (b) changing from white bread to wholewheat bread;
    (c) reducing added sugar to drinks and cereals;
    (d) avoiding processed and tinned vegetables and fruit;
    (e) reducing the consumption of soft drinks;
    (f) experimenting with other forms of sweeteners – i.e. honey, fruit, parsnips, molasses.

Fats – general

Fats are the major source of calories in the diet and are an essential ingredient for many of our tissues and cells. The basic building blocks of fats are the carbon atom (C) and the hydrogen atom (H). Fats are made up of a series of carbon atoms joined together in chains to which a number of hydrogen atoms are attached. If all the spaces around the carbon atom are filled, then the fat is said to be saturated. If only a few are filled, then it is unsaturated. Some fats are made up of a small number of carbon atoms (butter 4–18), whilst other have a long chain (beef fat 14–18).

```
    H   H   H   H              H       H           H
    |   |   |   |              |       |           |
H – C – C – C – C – H      H – C – C – C – C – C – C – C – C – H
    |   |   |   |                      |           |
    H   H   H   H                      H           H
```
Saturated Fat   *Unsaturated Fat*

Characteristics

Short chain fats	Liquid at room temperature
Long chain fats	Solid at room temperature
Saturated fats	Animal fat – solid at room temperature
(poly)unsaturated fats	Vegetable oils – liquid at room temperature

81

Cholesterol

This is a complex fatty substance made by the liver which is used by the body to form many essential substances (hormones – oestrogens – testosterone – bile salts). Everyone has a certain amount of cholesterol in their blood stream and in their diet. If the level of cholesterol is increased, then it is deposited along the walls of the arteries and causes partial blockage (much like the furring produced inside a kettle). It is this blockage of blood supply to the muscles of the heart that leads to heart attacks or to the brain that leads to strokes.

The important thing to realise about cholesterol is that it is an important and necessary part of the body's structure. However, as our diets have increased in their fatty content, the levels of cholesterol have become dangerously high and certainly predispose to the increased frequency of heart attacks and strokes.

Before entering the debate as to whether you should change from butter to margarine, it is important to point out that what is required is a reduction in the *total fat content* in the diet no matter what its source. This involves reducing the amount of fried food as well as such things as salad dressing, fatty cheese, eggs, pastries, chocolate, cream, nuts and red meats. Reducing the fat content in your diet to below 30% of the total calories may require you to reduce your meat intake. It is seldom possible to achieve this reduction whilst consuming a high red meat diet. Even lean cuts of meat contain as much as 25%–30% fat and a beef-steak is at least 45% fat. You would have to eliminate almost all other sources of fat including dairy products to achieve a diet less than 30% fat if you eat red meat. Finding sources of protein other than meat is an important factor in moving towards a more wholesome diet.

Butter or margarine

Many millions of pounds have been spent researching this question and even more money has been made by companies advertising the benefits of their particular product. Margarine and other vegetable sources of 'spreads' are a perfectly appropriate way of reducing the amount of saturated (animal source) fats in your diet. It is the saturated fats that appear to be more instrumental in producing atherosclerosis. However, if the total fat content in the diet remains the same, then the problems still arise. Therefore, if you can reduce your fat intake substantially then there is no requirement for you to switch from butter to margarine. However, if your fat content is the 'normal' high level present in the average diet (fried foods more than twice a week, meat more than three times a week, pastries and full fat cheese more than once a week) then you would be well advised to substitute a vegetable source of bread spread for butter.

Polyunsaturated fats are normally liquid at room temperatures. To make them solid and thus spreadable, manufacturers pass these substances through a complex chemical process called hydrogenation. This is a new and artificial process and the oils and fats so produced are a not naturally occurring product. It is wiser to use those oils which are the pure extracts of the vegetable or grain, i.e. olive oil, corn oil, sunflower oil, safflower oil, and to avoid the manufactured oils and spreads. Oils, including nuts, go rancid if left open or in the light and are not suitable for consumption. Similarly, heating oils above 375° seems to potentiate their ability to cause artherosclerosis which may explain the importance of reducing fried foods to a minimum.

Lecithin
Lecithin is another fatty derivative present in peas and beans but also made by the liver. It is a 'phospholipid' and aids in dissolving and emulsifying more complex forms of fat including cholesterol and the 'atheroma' present in the lining of the arteries. Lecithin can also be manufactured and has been used as an artificial additive to the diet.

Onion and garlic
It is interesting to note that both these substances appear to protect the body from the effects of a high fat diet and that many cultures where olive oil is used in the diet (Italy and Greece) have many recipes where raw onions and garlic are a basic ingredient to this 'high-fat' diet.

Reducing fat content in our diet involves:
  (1) Reduction in fried foods.
  (2) Changing from red meats to chicken, fish or dairy source of protein.
  (3) Increasing beans and 'sprouts' as sources of protein.
  (4) Reducing bread spreads of whatever variety.
  (5) Changing from fatty cheese to cottage cheese.
  (6) Changing from full cream milk to skimmed milk.

Proteins

Our total content of protein has not altered over many centuries. However, the source of protein has. Most people equate protein with meat and believe that other sources of protein are somehow 'second class'. This is wrong. The image of the prize-fighter eating steaks for breakfast is not one which is basic to a healthy diet. Another popular misconception is to confuse a meat-less diet with being a vegetarian. Some of the more unhealthy diets are those where individuals have given up eating meat but not made the necessary changes to produce balanced meals. We are not specifically focussing on the moral or economic issues relating to food, but there are increasingly good reasons why we should question our high intake of meat that are not specifically dietary. The technology of 'protein production' in the form of battery chickens, force-feeding, hormone stimulation, and anti-biotic prescribing is particularly concerning. As a nation we consume more than our fair share of the world's protein – and on average it takes 7–9 times the amount needed to produce one ton of animal protein as it does to produce a non-animal form of protein (beans, grains, rice). Yet, these foods contain more than sufficient quantity of protein to make up a balanced diet.

What is a protein?

Proteins are the 'building bricks' and 'skeleton' of the body. They form the basic structures of the muscles, bones and other tissues. A high protein diet is required at times of growth (childhood, pregnancy) when new structures are being created. Proteins are made of a series of 'amino acids' joined together and, like carbohydrates and fats, contain both carbon and hydrogen atoms. Proteins also contain the nitrogen atom, which is the difference between them and the other two basic constituents of our diet. Proteins are not a usual source of calories or energy and are essential ingredients for other reasons.

Sources of protein

Meat, fish	Grains
Milk, cheese, eggs	Nuts
Legumes (beans)	Sprouted seeds

For many cultures, meat and fish are not the normal source of protein and it is possible to obtain a perfectly adequate amount of protein by eating a combination of grains and beans. Most of the traditional diets in non-westernised cultures have a staple diet of these two ingredients; India – dahl and rice; America – chowder peas and corn bread; England – bread and cheese. Some wheats contain up to 14% protein, although the average is about 7%. Beans are a particularly good source of protein but have unfortunately gone out of fashion. If you are going to reduce your meat intake, try not to substitute just dairy foods. Experiment with bean dishes. Some people find beans produce too much gas and cause discomfort as well as social embarrassment. Beans can be 'de-gassed' by allowing them to soak well and changing the water at least once. They should then be rinsed well before cooking and should never be cooked in the water they have been soaked in.

Guidelines to protein consumption
(a) Reduce or eliminate red meat consumption.
(b) Eat fish, chicken or cheese.
(c) Introduce a bean dish once a week.

Vegetables and Fruits
One of the major changes in our diets has been a general reduction in the consumption of vegetables, especially the leafy green variety. Of the vegetables we do eat, a higher proportion are refined, processed or frozen. The importance of vegetables and fruits in the diet is that they provide an excellent source of the vitamins we require, especially vitamin B and vitamin C. The problem is that soaking and prolonged cooking destroy these vitamins. The one addition to everyone's kitchen should be a steamer. Steaming vegetables not only preserves the vitamins, the vegetables retain their taste. Fruit and vegetables provide a major source of 'fibre' to the diet whether eaten raw or cooked. Eating raw vegetables requires proper chewing and limits the quantity that can be consumed. One should aim towards eating at least three portions of leafy green vegetables a week (greens, broccoli, kale, spinach). Fruit should be washed and preferably peeled before eating.

Fibre
Fibre is being reinstated into our diet and at the moment is receiving a 'good press'. Fibre is sometimes called roughage, whereas its effect on the bowel suggests that it should be called

softage. Fibre is that part of the diet that is not absorbed by the body. Because it was not considered an essential component until its reinstatement a few years ago, the fibre content of our diet had reduced ten-fold.

TABLE V

Fibre

Cellulose Lignins	}	Vegetables
Gums Pectins Mucilage	}	Fruit

'Fibre' is made up of a number of different constituents as shown in Table V. It provides bulk to the stool and decreases the 'intestinal-transit time'. This means that a person on a low fibre diet evacuates a meal 72 hours after eating, whilst someone on a high fibre diet evacuates the same meal in under forty hours. Because fibre adds bulk to the motion, it aids in defecation and the pressure required to open one's bowels is reduced.

TABLE VI

Conditions thought to be associated with low fibre diet

Appendicitis
Gall bladder disease
Obesity
Diabetes
Constipation
Diverticulitis
Large bowel cancer
Haemorrhoids
Varicose veins
Hiatus hernia

As can be seen from the list of conditions associated with a low fibre diet in Table VI, the adage 'an apple a day keeps the doctor away' is perfectly true. Adding fibre (bran) to the diet can be an easy way of combating this deficiency. Changing from white bread to wholewheat bread, eating high-fibre cereals, or fruits and vegetables are an even better way.

Vitamins

Since the discovery of vitamins seventy years ago, scientists and nutritionists have been influenced by the notion that one vitamin deficiency causes one disease – e.g. low vitamin C causes scurvy. Whereas this is undoubtedly true, it is important to appreciate that it is possible to arrive at vitamin deficiency without having the obvious clinical signs of deficiency and that extra vitamin supplement may be required during special circumstances. Thus it is well understood that during pregnancy extra iron and calcium may be needed.

There are many individuals who feel that extra vitamins are required during stressful periods or after recovery from an illness. Whether high doses of vitamin C actually prevent colds is still much debated. Generally speaking, additional vitamin supplements are not necessary if the diet is well balanced and derived from good fresh produce. Too many people 'pop' vitamin pills and assume they are keeping to a health diet. More often than not they are by-passing the need to take a good look at their diet and to become more involved in the cooking and eating of it. We are always looking for short cuts. Much as it may seem sensible, vitamin supplementing is not a good way of ensuring a healthy diet. Nevertheless, there are occasions and diseases not normally associated with vitamin deficiency when additional supplements are essential.

Minerals and trace elements

The importance of minerals and trace elements in the diet has been for too long disregarded by the medical profession. Fortunately this is now changing and we are becoming more aware of the importance of these minute quantities in our diet. The body does not store minerals in any great quantity and they need to be constantly replenished through the diet. Recently hair analysis has been suggested as a way of determining whether there are trace-mineral deficiencies. The accuracy of some of the commercial firms, measuring the mineral content of hair, has been called into question and the test is not sufficiently accurate for it to be used as a diagnostic. However, it can be used as a useful 'screening test' and if any deficiencies are highlighted, more complicated and expensive tests are available – but usually only as research procedures.

VITAMIN	Food Source	Function	Deficiency Symptoms
Vitamin A (carotene)	Green vegetables, milk, cream cheese, fish liver oil, liver, kidney.	Essential for growth, health of the eyes, structure and functioning of the skin and mucous membrane.	Night blindness, low resistance to infection, infection of mucous membrane, i.e. catarrh, bronchial complaints. Skin and nervous tissue disorders.
Vitamin B1 (thiamine)	Yeast, wheat germ, kelp, soya beans, green vegetables, milk, eggs, oysters, meat and liver.	Essential for growth, carbohydrate metabolism and function of the heart, nerves and muscles.	Nervous disorders, blood disorders, skin and hair problems, depression, beri-beri, gastric disorders, ulcers.
Vitamin B2 (riboflavine)	Yeast, wheat germ, soya beans, peanuts, green vegetables, milk, eggs, meat, fowl.	Essential for growth, health of hair and mouth, general well-being, function of eyes.	Dry hair and skin, retarded or slow growth, mouth and tongue sores, poor vision, nervous disorders, lack of staminia.
Vitamin B3 (pantothenic acid)	Yeast, liver, eggs, brown rice, bran,	Health of skin and hair. Essential for	Dry skin and hair.

VITAMIN	Food Source	Function	Deficiency Symptoms
Vitamin B6 (pyridoxine)	whole grain products. Yeast, wheat germ, melon, cabbage, milk, egg yolk, fish.	growth of all tissue. Protein metabolism. Health of skin. Function of nerves and muscles.	Skin eruptions, nervous rashes, irritability, insomnia, muscle cramps.
Vitamin B12 (cyanocobalamine)	Yeast, spinach, lettuce, eggs, liver, meat.	Health of nerve tissue and skin. Protein metabolism.	Anaemia, tiredness, skin disorders, poor appetite.
Biotin	Liver, kidney, vegetables, nuts.	Probably necessary for healthy skin, function of nerves, muscles and mucous membranes.	Undetermined.
Choline	Egg yolk, liver, kidney, brains, sweetbreads, dried yeast.	Essential for the functioning of the liver. Prevent build-up of fatty acids.	Premature ageing. Build-up of fatty acids.
Folic acid	Green leafy vegetables, liver, brewer's yeast.	Important for red blood cell formation, for growth and division of cells.	Poor growth, anaemia, vitamin B12 deficiency.

VITAMIN	Food Source	Function	Deficiency Symptoms
PABA (para-aminobenzoic acid)	Liver, yeast, wheat germ, molasses.	Aids bacteria in forming folic acid; aids red blood cell formation.	Fatigue, irritability, depression, constipation.
Inositol	Eggs, meat, liver, kidney, whole grain products.	Essential for the functioning of the liver. Prevents build-up of fatty acids.	Premature ageing. Build-up of fatty acids.
Niacin (nicotinic acid, nicotinamide)	Yeast, liver, kidney, milk, whole grain products; and can be converted by the body from tryptophan.	Essential for growth, health of skin, function of the stomach and intestines and nerves.	Pellagra, skin disorders, nervous and intestinal disturbances, headaches, insomnia.
Vitamin C (ascorbic acid)	Citrus fruits, melon, berries, tomatoes, raw vegetables.	Essential for growth, cell activity, health of gums and teeth.	Sore gums, lack of immunity to infection, pains in joints, scurvy.
Vitamin D	Milk, butter, fish, liver oil, eggs, fresh green vegetables, sunshine.	Formation of bones and teeth, regulating calcium and phosphorus metabolism.	Tooth decay, bone deformities, calcium and phosphorus deficiency, rickets.

VITAMIN	Food Source	Function	Deficiency Symptoms
Vitamin E (tocopherol)	Seed germ oils, egg yolks, green vegetables, milk.	Normal reproduction. Function of nerves, muscles.	Premature ageing, incomplete pregnancies, sterility in males, muscular and nervous disorders.
Vitamin F (fatty acids)	Safflower, soya, corn and cod liver oil.	Helps regulate blood coagulation and is essential for normal glandular activity.	Brittle hair and nails, dandruff, varicose veins.
Vitamin K	Soya beans, vegetable oils, green leafy vegetables, tomatoes, liver.	Essential for blood clotting.	Prolonged bleeding from cuts and sores, lack of clotting agent.

SOME ESSENTIAL TRACE ELEMENTS IN THE BODY AND THEIR IMPORTANCE

Mineral	Importance	Deficiency symptoms	Suggested dietary allowance per day	Source
Cobalt	Is part of vitamin B12. Maintains red blood cells.	Pernicious anaemia.	Average daily intake is usually 5.0–8.0 mcg.	Liver, kidney, oysters and milk.
Copper	Necessary to formation of red blood cells. Is part of many enzymes.	Weakness, skin sores.	2 mg for adults.	Liver, whole grain products, green leafy vegetables.
Iodine	Necessary for proper function of the thyroid gland. Prevents goitre. Regulates body metabolism.	Enlarged thyroid. Loss of energy, dry skin and hair.	Men – 130 mcg. Women – 100 mcg.	Plant and animal seafoods.
Iron	Necessary for haemoglobin production. Promotes growth.	Anaemia, weakness, constipation.	Women – 18 mg. Men – 10 mg.	Leafy green vegetables, liver, dried apricots, walnuts.
Zinc	Necessary for insulin synthesis and male reproductive fluid. Aids healing process.	Retarded growth, delayed sexual maturity.	15 mg.	High protein diets, brewer's yeast, wheat bran, wheat germ.

THE MACRO-MINERALS OF THE BODY AND THEIR IMPORTANCE

Mineral	Importance	Deficiency symptoms	Suggested dietary allowance per day	Sources
Calcium	Necessary for strong bones and teeth. Helps normal blood clotting, muscle, nerve and heart functions.	Soft or brittle bones; back and leg pains.	0.8–1.4 grams depending on age.	Milk, dairy products, bone meal, calcium lactate.
Chlorine	Regulates acidity/alkalinity of the body. Helps produce digestive acids.	Loss of hair and teeth. Poor digestion.		Salt.
Magnesium	Helps the body to use fats, carbohydrates, protein and other nutrients.	Nervousness, tremors.	Men – 350 mg. Women – 300 mg.	Fresh green vegetables, soyabeans, corn, apples, almonds.

THE MACRO-MINERALS OF THE BODY AND THEIR IMPORTANCE

Mineral	Importance	Deficiency symptoms	Suggested dietary allowance per day	Sources
Phosphorus	Helps with calcium to build bones and teeth.	Loss of weight and appetite.	800 mg.	Fish, eggs, poultry, whole grain, nuts, meat.
Potassium	Helps control the activity of the nerves, kidneys and heart muscles.	Respiratory and heart failure.	Probably about 2 grams.	Leafy vegetables, oranges, whole grain, mint leaves, potato skins.
Sodium	Necessary for functioning of nerves, muscles, blood and the lymph system.	Weak or shrinking muscles. Loss of appetite, nausea.	6–18 grams, as sodium chloride (salt).	Salt, seafoods, beets, kelp, meat.
Sulphur	For the formation of body tissues.		Sufficient sulphur is obtained from normal protein intake.	Meat, fish, nuts, eggs, cabbage, Brussels sprouts.

Stimulants

Many of us will use food or drink as a way of cheering ourselves up or decreasing our anxiety. Usually the first thing we do in times of stress or crisis is to make a cup of tea or have a stiff drink. Coffee, tea and cocoa all contain active chemicals (caffeine, theophylline and theobromine) which are absorbed into the bloodstream and act like a stimulant. Their chemical structure is not dissimilar to that of adrenaline, the body's own stimulant. People who drink more than two cups of coffee or four cups of tea a day will have circulating levels of chemicals in their bloodstream which will maintain their level of arousal at a higher level than normal. It is like rearranging the thermostat on your boiler so that it switches off at a higher temperature. Maintaining an artificially high level of arousal will reduce your ability to cope with any additional stress and will keep your body/mind in a perpetual 'fight' response. When coffee and tea are reduced you may well feel lethargic and slow for a few days or even develop a 'coffee withdrawal' headache. It is nevertheless wise to reduce the coffee intake to below two cups a day and tea to four cups. This can allow you to experiment with other forms of fluid intake – fruit juices or herb tea. Herb teas – mint, hibiscus, camomile, rose-hip, lemon balm – all have an effect on the body and are indeed used by herbalists as medicines. Learning about their beneficial effects can be one of the pleasant surprises as you fight your coffee addiction.

More powerful addictions include the drugs (speed, glue solvents, cocaine, LSD, heroin) and it is obvious from the tragic results that they play no part in a holistic diet.

Alcohol/tobacco

These are the two more acceptable forms of drug addiction which nevertheless cause intense misery, disease and suffering for many individuals and families. There are as always no hard and fast rules and each person must develop their own guidelines.

It is generally accepted that smoking, however little, is harmful, causing lung cancer, duodenal ulcer and making bronchitis/emphysema much worse. If you have never smoked, don't start. If you smoke a little on occasion, give it up. If you are a regular heavy smoker, think hard about why you smoke and when you are certain you want to give it up, seek help. If you are over sixty and have smoked for many years, try reducing the amount you smoke, changing to low-tar brands and cutting ½–1" off each cigarette before you smoke. When trying to give up a 'bad habit', whatever it is, avoid 'guilt' or 'punishment' as incentives. Try and replace the 'bad habit' with a 'good habit' – walking or reading or a relaxation exercise.

Alcohol is not always 'bad' and on occasions can be positively beneficial. Surprising as it may seem, it is not a stimulant but a depressant on the nervous system. It 'blocks out' and anaesthetises thoughts and feelings as well as movements and speech. It releases people from their inhibitions and this may appear to excite and stimulate. Taken occasionally and moderately it does no harm. Taken frequently and in large quantities it becomes the most devastating drug present in our culture today – destroying more families than all the 'hard drugs' put together.

Food additives

The manufacturing and process of food has developed into a vast industry, and 'nutritional science' has become no more than an extension of chemical technology. Many of the additives in our food are there not for nutritional purposes but to ensure a commercially viable product. We the consumer are as much to blame and if we insist on having bread which is 'soft' and does not develop a mould after seven days – or want our apples to look red and 'apple-like' – then we cannot blame the food industry for producing these artificially created foods. The additives included in our food are:

Preservatives
These are added to prevent growth of bacteria and fungi. Preserving food has always been a challenge and it is possible to avoid the artificial additives with the sensible use of the refrigerator and other more traditional methods, such as vinegar in bread, herbs and spices for cooked meals. More important is to shop more frequently and eat fresh fruit and vegetables the same day.

Permitted colourings
Most of the ones used are of natural origin, but nevertheless they are only added for cosmetic reasons. Many sweets are artificially coloured and there is strong evidence to link these additives to the 'hyperactive child' syndrome.

Anti-oxidants
These are used to prevent fats going rancid and as a spray on apples and pears. Without them shelf-life of manufactured foods would be greatly reduced.

Chemical oxidisers
These are used in white bread to increase the 'whiteness' and stiffen the dough. The original chemical used (agene) had to be discontinued when it was discovered it produced nervous disorders in dogs.

Softeners
These again are used in white bread to produce the 'soft springy loaf'.

Emulsifiers and stabilisers
These are used to 'tenderise' cooked meats and to bind food ingredients together and avoid crumbling in cake mixes.

Modified starch
This is used to add bulk to food products.

Antibiotics/hormones
These are not usually considered as additives, but most of our poultry and cattle are given doses of antibiotics to prevent infection that arises because they are housed in overcrowded accommodation, and hormones to increase their bulk. Traces of these antibiotics and hormones are easily detectable in the meat we buy.

From January 1986 all foods will have to have all the additives marked on the packaging. It is quite a chore, however, to keep checking each item. Far more sensible is to buy fresh food and avoid tinned or packaged food. Visit your local health food store and see what substitutes you can purchase there.

Foods to combat the effects of stress

(1) Low-fat cultured dairy foods (cottage cheese, yogurt, buttermilk, kefir) provide protein and calcium.
(2) Nutritional yeast (try mixing it in juice) provides protein and B complex.

(3) Wheat germ provides protein, B complex, and essential oils.

(4) Soy products provide protein, essential oils, calcium, and potassium.

(5) Fresh fruit (particularly bananas, oranges and cantaloupe) provides potassium and vitamin C.

(6) Dried fruit provides potassium.

(7) Dark, green leafy vegetables provide vitamin A and C, calcium and iron.

Basic guidelines to a healthy diet

(1) Limit sugar intake (this means reading labels carefully); although canned foods, bottled sauces, dressings and cereals may sometimes be described as 'natural', they often contain high quantities of sugar.

(2) Avoid highly processed foods with preservatives and colouring added.

(3) Eat natural, whole grain breads, cereals, pasta and rice, rather than highly processed varieties.

(4) Eat plenty of fresh fruits and vegetables, rather than those which are frozen or canned.

(5) Eat high quality protein sources (low-fat dairy products, whole grains, beans, fish, eggs, fowl) and avoid high-fat meat, high-fat cheese, red meat, and processed meats.

(6) Find suitable beverages to replace coffee, tea and fizzy canned drinks. Try a variety of juices and drink plenty of spring water.

(7) Reduce salt intake by avoiding added salt and snack foods.

(8) Keep tobacco and alcohol consumption to a minimum and avoid unnecessary medication.

(9) Keep fast-food and canteen eating to the minimum.

(10) Reduce fried foods both at home and in restaurants. Cook vegetables in a steamer rather than a saucepan.

(11) Try to eat your largest meal in the earlier part of the day to ensure the body is able to rest more at night.

(12) Give yourself time to eat slowly, peacefully, and with concentration. That way you will be aware when you have eaten enough and will be less likely to over-eat. Digestion is aided by a peaceful mind and body.

6

UNDER- STANDING YOUR MIND

The title of this chapter is an immediate indication of the difficulty we face when approaching the area of the mind. For how can we study the mind when we use the mind to study it? This problem has taxed philosophers, thinkers and theologians throughout the ages, and the study of the mind in reality encompasses the study of mankind. In a short chapter we can only attempt to outline the various directions in which man has travelled in the study of the mind and will limit our descriptions to those areas that relate in some way to the other chapters. We shall focus on some fairly practical aspects as they affect daily living and trust that in simplifying this immensely complex subject we will retain some valuable information and provide some useful exercises.

Models of the mind

We take it for granted that our mind is in some way linked with our brain and if it resides anywhere it must be somewhere in our head. In fact, this is a relatively recent notion, for the Egyptians believed that mind-spirit-soul resided not in the brain but in the bowels and heart. The Sumerians thought it resided in the liver and even the great philosopher Aristotle saw the heart as the seat of thought and feeling. Aristotle and Plato, his teacher, were the major Western philosophers whose opinions concerning the mind held sway right from 300 BC until the sixteenth and seventeenth centuries. Even now, the study of the mind is hampered by the descriptions outlined thousands of years ago by these two great men. Their observations were a great step forward, but because of their greatness few individuals had the courage to build on their descriptions. The relationship between Plato and Aristotle is beautifully expressed in Raphael's majestic fresco 'The School of Athens'. There we see Plato, with hand upraised pointing to the stars, whereas Aristotle, holding a copy of Plato's book *Timaeus*, is pointing to the earth. Although Plato is seen as a great rationalist, he did not believe in trusting the senses and arrived at his great description of the mind, knowledge and civilisation through a mixture of mystical contemplation and mathematics. Plato's *Republic* gives a description as to how he saw the perfect civilisation. The outline is based on an oligarchy (government by the few) and Plato's ideas are relatively hierarchical. Because he valued reason above all other attributes, it followed that it should reside in the topmost part of the body – the head. Plato felt knowledge was better acquired not from observation but through 'vision of truth', and the parable of 'the cave' is his clearest description of how man is entrapped and chained by his limited visions. Aristotle was far more of a realist then Plato and was himself a great biologist. It is ironic that he felt the heart to be the seat of life – the soul and mind – and the brain function was to cool the blood that carried the life-force through the body. However, although Aristotle's observations were inaccurate, they were balanced by his foundation of the system of deductive logic which still governs the principles of rational debate to this day. Both Plato and Aristotle were instrumental in seeing the mind's chief faculty as reason and logic, and the early Christian church incorporated some aspects of their philosophies. The early church had a major influence in maintaining the notion that mind, spirit and soul were all closely linked, and to some extent this gave church leaders a certain control over not only the study of the mind but what the mind should think, feel and imagine. The persecution of the witches and the tortures of the Inquisition were justified because the victims of these activities showed obvious signs of deranged minds. Even though Hippocrates in the fifth century BC had suggested that epilepsy was a physical disorder, nevertheless many sufferers were subjected to purges, incantations and sacrifices and were seen to be possessed by the Devil. For the church, a healthy mind meant believing in its dogma and an unhealthy mind meant allying oneself with the forces of evil.

It took another two great men to free man from the grip of the church. Leonardo Da Vinci, who insisted on studying the body through dissection and not simply through inference and intuition, described the brain with its hemispheres and ventricles and laid the foundation for modern neuroanatomy.

Descartes, whom we mentioned in the first chapter, brought together the principles which established the importance of the mind, separate both from the body and the soul. Newton provided the basis for the scientific method by highlighting the power of ration-or-reason, as Aristotle had done earlier. As a result of their studies, the *dualistic* (separating mind from matter-body), *mechanistic* (regarding the body, including the brain, as a machine) and *reductionistic* (reducing things to their smallest components) modes of thought and behaviour became the prevalent model or pair of spectacles that have held sway right up until moderm times. Although much of this book is challenging the limitations of this model, we must not forget how much is owed to those great men.

From the seventeenth century onwards, the study of the mind was in some way overshadowed by the study of the body and it is not until the late nineteenth and early twentieth century that further steps were taken to understanding the workings of the mind.

Psychoanalysts, Psychologists, Psychiatrists

Psychoanalysts	Followers of Freud, may or may not be doctors
Psychologists	Study workings of the mind, not doctors
Psychiatrists	Doctors treating mental disorders, usually drugs
Psychotherapists	Doctors or non-doctors who treat mental disorders without drugs

Sigmund Freud stands out as one of the great innovators in the study of the mind. He studied medicine and neurology and was initially influenced by Breuer, who used hypnosis to release painful memories in cases of hysteria. Many of the patients Freud saw in Vienna were heavily influenced by the social prohibitions on sexual matters. It appeared to Freud that the painful memories released, first through hypnosis and then through 'free association', invariably contained a sexual content.

He reintroduced the concept of 'energy' into the workings of the mind and labelled this energy 'libido'. He went on to describe two models of the mind which still form the basis of much psychoanalytic thinking. The first divided the mind into *conscious, preconscious* and *unconscious*. The conscious part of the mind contains all immediately accessible information and memories of present and past experiences. The preconscious contains those memories that with an effort of will we can recall, and the unconscious is the repository of all that is forgotten or repressed, and, Freud felt, other painful events. Psychoanalysis is the process by which we can make the unconscious material available to our conscious mind. Freud thought that as long as important events remained unconscious, the mind would remain limited in its capabilities and primitive in its behaviour. The second model of the mind included the *ego* (conscious part, aware of the self), *super-ego* (judging critical part influenced by parents, teachers, priests) and *id* (unconscious, childlike, primitive part). Freud saw psychoanalysis as a means of strengthening the *ego* and releasing it from the influences of the *super-ego* and *id*. It is interesting that Freud's second description of the mind fits well with that of the Huna culture and with most people's everyday experience of themselves, i.e. we have a *higher* self that tells, guides, judges, criticises, leads and directs us; a *middle* self which is the way we operate on an everyday practical basis, and a *lower* self which contains our instincts, drives, uncontrolled urges and habit patterns. The study of the mind therefore was the study of how Colonel Super-ego, Lieutenant Ego and Private Id got on together. Freud called the language used by the ego and super-ego 'secondary process' and that used by id 'primary process', which included the language of dreams, slips of the tongue, free association. Freud felt that the balance between super-ego, ego and id was heavily influenced by the early experiences provided by the parents and that the mind was shaped and moulded by the relationships between father, mother and infant.

Many of Freud's followers have since altered and added to his theories, but his fundamental descriptions of the unconscious elements in the mind still stand as his major achievement and retain their influence to this day. Jung, initially Freud's closest follower, described a very separate area in the workings of the mind. He felt that not only did the mind have a *personal unconscious* as a result of the individual's early experiences, but that the mind was also influenced by *collective* unconscious. By that he meant that the mind had access to and was influenced by all the collective memories of the race, culture, society, nation to which that individual belonged. Freud dismissed this idea as fanciful and unscientific, but again, like Freud's own discoveries, it links well with several older descriptions of the mind. The fascination we have for myths, legend, folklore, fairy stories, parables and rituals indicate the links between the personal mind and the collective mind. Jung studied these collective experiences and described in detail how he felt the individual mind was shaped by them. He compared these collective experiences in different cultures and was able to identify recurring themes, such as the hero myth (Ulysses, Robin Hood).

Between them Freud and Jung discovered, like the voyagers of old, new territories in the mind, the personal and the collective unconscious.

A totally different line of enquiry was followed by the early psychologists who treated the mind as if it were a physical entity, linked entirely to the workings of the brain. This group of psychologists were known as *behavioural psychologists* because they felt the appropriate way to study the mind was to study how it affected the behaviour of the individual. They applied the scientific measuring instruments used in other disciplines to help determine how the mind functioned. They saw the mind as being influenced by 'conditioning'. The mind responded to a stimulus (food), by a response (eating). The response was either rewarded (hunger assuaged) or punished (feeling sick). Skinner, the most eminent of this group, believed that all behaviour could be explained by the various permutations and combinations of this simple sequence.

The classical experiments by Pavlov illustrated this scientifically: Pavlov rang bells and gave dogs food at the same time. He found that after a while, he would ring the bells and the dogs would salivate even though no food was present.

For Skinner, all phenomena of the mind could be explained through the science of behaviourism, and in the most extreme form of this theory he maintained that 'free will' was an illusion described by idealists who refused to accept the proofs of his discoveries. Behavioural psychology has led to treating mental disturbances as if they were inappropriate conditioned responses. If you are afraid of flying, the mental responses to entering an aeroplane have nothing to do with your past early experience or, if they do, it is irrelevant to subsequent treatment. The individual with a fear is gradually introduced to the stimulus (aeroplane) and is rewarded every time he is able to reduce his fear or punished if his response is 'wrong'. Behavioural psychologists introduced a new and important dimension to the study of the mind which appeared to be in total opposition to that of the analysts, and certainly their methods of treating mental disorders were very different.

The next group of psychologists who studied the mind were the *humanistic psychologists*. This group felt that it was unhelpful to reduce the mind to the Freudian mental structure of super-ego, ego and id, or the experimental processes of operant conditioning described by Skinner and his followers. They felt these 'models' somehow did not describe the essential experience of being human. They looked to existential philosophers for their inspiration. Maslow, a major writer in this area, outlined the need the mind has for reaching its full potential through creative acts.

Humanistic psychologists studied the workings of the mind by studying especially creative or gifted people. They emphasised the healthy aspects of the mind and laid the foundation to the 'positive thinking' school. Think positively and you will behave positively. They emphasised the strength of the conscious mind and its ability to overcome the *unconscious* influences. Therapists trained in this model of the mind limit the exploration of 'unconscious tendencies' and do not expose their clients to controlled behaviour modification. They tend to focus on the enhancement of the individual's emotional life and reinforce the positive and healthy tendencies already present. They focus on the 'here and now' rather than the past or future.

Psychiatrists who use drugs or ECT (electroconvulsive therapy, which is electrical stimulation of the brain) to manage mental disorders see the mind, like the behaviourists, as a function of the brain. The brain is like other organs in the body and can be studied using the instruments that doctors have used to study other organs. They have been influenced therefore by the neuroanatomists and neurophysiologists who have studied the brain and the mind with increasing success in the last twenty to thirty years.

For centuries, men have drilled holes in the skull, probed and explored the brain using surgical and, more recently, electrical instruments. In the last thirty years brain surgeons have severed connections in the brain in an attempt to cure epilepsy and portions of the brain have been removed to treat personality disorders.

In more recent years, the electroencephalograph (EEG) has been used to measure electrical activity arising from the brain and, as with a jig saw puzzle, the link between the anatomical parts of the brain and its functions is slowly being discovered. For the purposes of this book we shall limit ourselves to a description of the mental functions of the brain and the way they influence our daily life. The major part of the brain is made up of two hemispheres joined by millions of neurons (nerve cells with long connecting threads). The left hemisphere controls the movement on the right side of the body and the right hemisphere controls the left side of the body. In addition, the left hemisphere governs those functions principally to do with speech, rational thought, logical reasoning, objective analysis, whilst the right hemisphere is concerned with how things relate to one another.

FUNCTIONS

		Left hemisphere	Right hemisphere
		Thoughts	Feeling
		Linear reason	Initiative
Corpus Callosum		Verbal	Non-verbal
		Objective	Subjective
		Mathematics	Images
		Literature	Patterns/ Shape
Left hemisphere	Right hemisphere	Extrovert	Introvert
		Reading	Rhythm
Neuron		Analysis	Synthesis

The right hemisphere recognises shapes, patterns and images, and it covers our intuitive sense. It appears that each hemisphere can function independently of the other, but that in most people one hemisphere plays a more dominant role. For most people the left hemisphere is the dominant hemisphere, resulting in more right-handed persons. Not only does the dominant hemisphere govern the movement and handedness but it seems to determine the prevailing 'consciousness' or mode of thought. A simple exercise to determine how you respond to 'both sides' is described by Ornstein to illustrate this.

> *Close your eyes and attempt to sense each side of your body separately. Try to get in touch with the feelings of the left and of the right side, their strengths and weaknesses. When you are finished, open your eyes for a moment and reflect on one of these questions. Close your eyes and sense inside for an answer, then repeat the process with the next question:*
> (1) *Which side of you is more feminine?*
> (2) *Which is more masculine?*
> (3) *Which do you consider the 'dark side' of yourself?*
> (4) *Which is more active?*
> (5) *Which side is more logical?*
> (6) *Which side is more artistic?*

The differences between the left and right side of our bodies and how we feel about them indicate in part the balance between the left and right hemispherical modes of consciousness. In other words, we have the capacity for two modes of mental functioning, each governed by a different part of our brain. Part of the conflict we experience inside ourselves and in our daily lives is an extension of the conflict that can occur between the functioning of the two hemispheres. Which one will be allowed to dominate – our thinking, rational mode (left hemisphere) or our feeling, intuitive mode (right hemisphere)? One could extend this description to include most of the conflicts that we see being acted out in the world today. Our culture is one that defines reality by creating opposites, e.g. masculine/feminine, good/evil, rich/poor, happy/unhappy, strong/weak. These opposite polarities need each other. How can we have a quality of happiness if there is no quality of unhappiness, how can there be a 'rich' person if there are no 'poor' persons? These polarities are often seen in opposition to each other – good must fight evil, a healthy person is 'better' than a sick person. In fact, the mind, because of its two methods of consciousness, accentuates the differences and helps maintain the conflict between the polarities.

It is only in the last twenty years that we have begun to understand the working of the mind from this perspective and it has allowed many individuals to become aware of the potential not only in the less dominant hemisphere (usually the right) but in the 'wisdom' that arises when both hemispheres operate not in conflict but in harmony. Creating a balance in our mental life may require us to increase the functioning of our less dominant hemisphere and then balance the activity from each side. A good analogy is that of a stereo system as shown in the diagrams. When both speakers are balanced (see diagram), the stereo effect is greater than the sum of the two speakers.

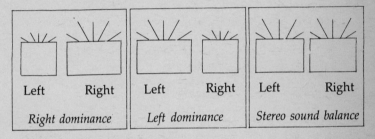

Left Right	Left Right	Left Right
Right dominance	*Left dominance*	*Stereo sound balance*

Products of the mind

Another way of understanding your mind is to examine what it produces, and how these 'products' themselves affect the working of the mind. The first 'product' of the mind that we have already alluded to throughout this book is the capacity for awareness, or consciousness.

Consciousness

This has been variously defined by the differing groups of people who have studied it from poets to psychologists and mystics. As we have already intimated, it is not a static phenomenon. If it is defined as 'that of which one is aware', then it will alter from moment to moment and be influenced by a complex set of factors both internal and external. The capacity for increasing our awareness will determine the state of our consciousness. Consciousness can be compared to the 'pair of spectacles' through which we perceive our reality, and our perceptions will in turn affect our consciousness. If I put on a pair of blue spectacles, all will appear blue: as I perceive all things blue, this reinforces my belief that there is only a 'blue reality'. This will in turn limit my awareness (consciousness) of any 'not-blue' items. If someone wearing a yellow pair of spectacles comes along, the likelihood of our agreeing as to how the world is determined is fairly small.

Conflicts between people often occur because their capacity for awareness is different and from their own perspective they are 'right' and the other person is 'wrong'. It is this transitory and arbitrary aspect of consciousness that led the eastern philosophers to label reality as 'an illusion'. They developed a method by which they were able to alter their state of consciousness and thus their capacity of awareness. They called this process *meditation* and we shall describe this skill in detail at the end of this chapter. The state of your consciousness will affect the more well-defined products of your mind.

Influences on the mind

In the same way that walking on a broken leg will be painful and is likely to retard the healing process, it is important to be aware of how using your mind when it is distressed may be counter-productive. Before exploring ways of both 'resting' the mind and enhancing its capacities, it is important to remember the external factors that do influence its activity. They will have been described in greater detail in other chapters but we will remind you of them again.

Drugs – Alcohol – Coffee – Food

Drugs that affect the working of the mind are sometimes used by psychiatrists to treat mental distress from depression to anxiety. In addition, the epidemic of addictive drug abuse involving marijuana, heroin and cocaine indicates how prevalent and serious this effect of drugs on the mind has become. They are used to elevate mood and create a feeling of euphoria as well as to diminish anxiety and fearfulness. The large-scale use of tranquilisers is another indication of how reliant we have become on these artificial 'mind-benders'. Nevertheless, the most prevalent mood drug used is alcohol and although its abuse is increasing and the problems it produces are devastating for many people, it still serves as a useful and necessary additive to their daily life. This is equally true for coffee and tea and many people still do not appreciate how drinking these stimulant drinks will alter their mental life and affect the 'products of their mind'.

Even less well known is the fact that the ordinary food we eat has an effect on our mental life. Ayurvedic medicine, the traditional form of Indian medicine, paid great attention to this aspect of food. The doctors trained in this system described how some foods (meat, spices) elevated mood and created a more aggressive mental state; some foods (dairy products, fatty foods) depressed mood and helped create a more passive, depressed state; whilst still others (beans, rice, vegetables) helped produce a clear, balanced, integrated mental state. They would prescribe a 'diet' according to the symptoms of the patient and, like Hippocrates, they made food their drugs and not drugs their food.

Finally, in more recent times, we have had to cope with the numerous additives that are now present in many of our food substances. Their effect on the mind is still debated, but many more nutritionists now recognise their potential for mood change.

The *physical state of the body*, including tension and breathing pattern, all helps to determine the state of the mind, and the much repeated phrase 'a healthy body means a healthy mind' is not just a cliché. The breathing pattern is probably the most important physical aspect affecting the mind and we have outlined this in much greater detail elsewhere.

The *physical state of the environment* has been well known to affect psychological states and our everyday experience is that we 'feel better' and are 'more alive' in certain geographical situations, e.g. by the seaside, on a mountain, in the countryside. Conversely, stuffy, artificially lit environments can affect people, adversely producing headaches or feelings of stuffiness, lethargy and depression. Certain 'winds' or air masses that occur usually before a thunder storm affect a large number of people, making them more nervous and irritable. The cause seems to be the level of 'ionisation' in the atmosphere. Most air molecules are neutral and carry no electric charge. If the atmosphere contains more positive charged ions, as occurs in cities, in foggy conditions or before a storm, they in some way affect the mind and body to produce these commonly shared experiences. Air which contains more negative ions, as occurs by the seaside or on top of a mountain, is felt to be 'invigorating', 'bracing' and more relaxing. One of the reasons for suggesting a 'change' or holiday to someone who is stressed may result from the recognition that the atmosphere is not right in some way. Certain people appear to be more sensitive to atmospheric conditions than others and can be quite severely affected by sudden changes. The use of ionisers to change the ionisation of the atmosphere has been introduced to good effect in several institutions.

Social, cultural and racial factors are obviously of great importance as external influences on the mind. The way an Englishman thinks about a certain situation will be different from the way an Algerian or Indian thinks. There will of course be similarities, but the 'collective' nature of the 'Englishness' or 'Indianness' will determine the state of awareness each possesses and thus the perceptions each forms. The differences often surface in the language of each nationality – Eskimos have over seven different words for snow, obviously because in their environment the necessity to differentiate between one form of snow and another is much more important than it is for an Englishman. Because we have no other word for snow than snow, we can only think of snow in one way. It has been said that 'words put chains on thoughts' and it is not difficult to see how our cultural and national inheritance both shapes and limits our capacities for awareness.

Family, personal and past experiences for the most part help to shape the way 'the mind develops'. In the section on psychoanalysis we described how the unconscious portion of the mind is thought to influence the conscious, and many of our habit patterns, ways of thinking, values and judgements are influenced by our parents. Whilst as children we usually accept this direction without criticism, during adolescence there is a tendency to challenge and reject many of these parental influences. Adults are thought to have arrived at their own decisions concerning their perceptions of the world about them. Adults have discarded those values, judgements and ideas inherited from their parents with which they disagree and accepted those with which they agree. The extent they are still unconscious or unaware of these influences on their mental activity is the extent to which, using Plato's terms, they are 'still in the cave'. Much of modern therapy concerns itself with freeing individuals from the 'scripts' (patterns of thought and behaviour inherited from childhood).

Before proceeding to the next section, it would be useful to summarise what has been covered so far.

(1) Models of the mind

Neuroanatomy	*Psychoanalysis*
Left and right hemispheres with two modes of consciousness	Conscious/unconscious super-ego (parents)
	ego id
	(adult) (child)

MIND

Humanistic psychology	*Behavioural psychology*
Uniqueness of human experience – self-worth – positive emotions	Stimulus-response

(2) Influences on the mind

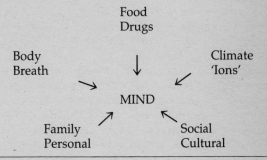

Food
Drugs

Body
Breath

Climate
'Ions'

MIND

Family
Personal

Social
Cultural

(3) Products of the mind

Consciousness	Dreams
Thoughts	Myths
Feelings	'Slips'
Imagination	Words
Fantasies	Science
Images	Language
Ideas	and show social and physical structures

With the help of the three outlines, we can describe ways in which we can work with our minds in the same way as we have described ways in working with our bodies.

7

WORKING WITH YOUR MIND

Increasing awareness

Our awareness is linked to either something within ourselves – a physical sensation, a thought or a feeling – or something outside ourselves – a noise, an object or a person. Exercise to increase our capacity to become aware of specific aspects of our experience can be developed from the few exercises outlined below. Meditation is a way of not only settling the mind, like relaxing the body, but of enhancing our capacity for awareness generally.

Exercise I – Increase awareness from without to within

Start by sitting back in your chair and looking around you. Say to yourself, 'I am aware of . . . my bookcase. I am aware of a car going past my window.' Continue this process, bringing other senses into play – 'I am aware of the sound of paper being shuffled' – allow your awareness to roam wherever it wishes to go, without judging or censoring its activity.

After a few minutes, close your eyes and turn your attention to any physical sensations – 'I am aware of my leg hurting' or 'pins and needles in my feet' – and feelings – 'I am aware of my wanting to stop this exercise', etc. Again, allow your awareness to roam as it will and keep repeating whatever comes into your consciousness. Practice this exercise regularly and you can develop a greater sense of the two worlds you live in – the external and the internal.

Exercise II – Focusing

In the last exercise, your attention was allowed to roam freely: in this exercise, your attention will be focused on one object.

Choose an object. It can be anything – a flower or piece of fruit, a favourite picture or simply a pen. Focus your eyes on the object and repeat in the same manner as the last exercise – 'I am aware of . . . the colour of the orange, I am aware of the texture or the pores on the skin'. Continue repeating the sentence 'I am aware – ' (to yourself, if you prefer not to repeat them out loud). If you find yourself losing your concentration, then gently bring your attention back to the object and start again.

Quietening the mind – Meditation

For most of us, distressing thoughts, feelings, worries about the past or future, are a major source of stress. We can find it difficult to switch our minds off and even when we sleep we may be disturbed by dreams or nightmares. Meditation is a way of quietening the mind and freeing it from these disturbing and distressing thoughts. Meditation is not a religion, nor will you loose your own religion if you start to meditate. You can be a devout Christian, an agnostic, a Buddhist or even an atheist and meditate. Meditation is not just resting, nor is it sleeping, although the benefit you get from regular meditation is often superior to sleeping. Meditation is not a hypnotic trance and you cannot be made to do anything against your will. Having described what meditation is not, we'd better describe what it is.

Meditation allows you to achieve a sense of mastery of your awareness, both closing it down and opening it wide. It can be compared to learning how to control the two dials on a radio. You can tune into different stations by turning one dial and can decrease or increase the volume by turning another. The technical phrase used by scientists is to describe meditation as a state of relaxed non-aroused physiological functioning. Scientists have discovered that during meditation, certain important changes occur in the body similar to those found in deeply relaxed individuals.

These changes include a slowing of the pulse, a lowering of blood-pressure, a decrease in the breathing rate and an increase in the flow of blood in the fingers and toes. At the same time there are changes which take place in the electrical activity of the brain which can be measured by the EEG. These changes show a more regular electrical activity during meditation called alpha rhythm. People who are asked about their experiences whilst their brain patterns show alpha rhythm report being peaceful, quiet and having a sense of timelessness much like the feelings we described in the first chapter when we discussed the 'spiritual' nature of our beings. During meditation, there is also a fall in the stress hormone cortisol, and another measure of stress, the level of lactic acid in the blood, is also reduced. People who meditate regularly show an increase in their psychological stability, they show less anxiety and report that they have a greater sense of control over their lives. Many patients have been able to stop taking tranquillisers and sleeping tablets through the regular practice of meditation. Indeed, you may find you need less sleep and that you have more energy available for your work or study.

Although meditation is often associated with yogis and eastern religions, there has been a strong tradition of meditative practices in western religions as well (e.g. St Ignatius of Loyola, the Desert Fathers, St Teresa of Avila). Christian meditative practices are of two main types. There are discursive methods, where the individual is asked to reflect on a quotation from the Bible. This has been called reflection or contemplation. There are also non-discursive methods of meditation that have been used over the centuries, such as the famous Jesus prayer or prayer of simplicity, where a series of words, such as 'Jesus Christ have mercy on me', is repeated over and over again. *The Way of the Pilgrim* (French, 1930) describes the experiences of a Russian priest who repeated the Jesus prayer regularly. In eastern religions there are also many different forms of meditation: some involve keeping the eyes open, some include repeating a few words called a mantra, and others, like in Buddhism, require the individual to answer 'unanswerable questions' called Koans, the most famous one being 'What is the sound of one hand clapping?'

The purpose of most methods of meditation is to free the mind from the 'cramp of conscious control' and allow it to operate in neutral gear. For most beginners, this can be a difficult notion to grasp, for if we want to do something successfully, our way is to try harder. 'Trying hard' to meditate is not likely to help you meditate. It is important to learn how to 'let go' or surrender to the deeper and quieter part of yourself.

Exercise III – Learning to meditate

It is necessary to put aside some time – 10–20 minutes rather early in the morning or before you go to sleep at night. Find a quite place in your home, preferably one where you will not be disturbed. It is helpful to keep the same place for meditation as this reinforces the habit. It also gives that place in your home a special significance. The next step is to find an appropriate chair. Meditation is best practised sitting up. Of course you can meditate lying down on your bed, but there is a greater likelihood of your falling asleep. Meditation is not sleeping – you should be alert and awake. However, there is nothing to stop you practising meditation to help you to go off to sleep. Choose a chair which is comfortable and which has a straight back. It is important not to slouch, although there is no reason why you should not support your back with a cushion or pillow. Keep your head, neck and trunk erect. If your feet do not reach the floor comfortably, put a small cushion underneath them. If you prefer to sit on the floor, find the most comfortable position for yourself and try to tilt your pelvis by placing a small cushion under your seat.

Close your eyes and place your hands just above your knees. Focus your attention on your breathing. Gradually deepen your breathing, with your diaphragm, allowing the inhalation to follow the exhalation. Spend a few minutes focussing on your breath. Take your attention to your forehead – relax the muscles of your forehead – relax the muscles of your eyes – relax the muscles of your face. Check that your jaw s not too tightly closed and that your tongue is lying smooth and easily in your mouth. Relax your shoulders – relax your hands and fingers – relax your chest and abdomen – relax your thighs, knees, ankles and feet. Bring your attention back to your breathing – *Pause* – allow the breath to become smooth and even.

Now as you breath in, place the word 'so' on your breath, silently, without moving your lips. As you breath out, place the word 'hum' on your outbreath, silently, without moving your lips.

Continue to breathe smoothly and evenly, repeating the sounds 'so' and 'hum' on your inhalation and exhalation. If any thoughts, worries or distractions come into your mind, allow them to come and then allow them to go, bringing your attention back to your breathing and the sounds 'so' and 'hum'.

Continue for another 5–10 minutes, repeating the sounds internally in unison with your breath. When you are about to stop, bring some feeling back into your fingers and toes. Take a few deeper breaths in and out and gently open your eyes.

Tips to deepen your meditation
(1) Do not eat or drink for up to half-an-hour before.
(2) Meditate in a group.
(3) Buy a meditation tape.
(4) Practise breathing exercise (alternate nostrils, Chapter 4).
(5) Avoid stimulant foods and alcohol.

Developing the right side of your brain
We described in the previous chapter how the right hemisphere of the brain is broadly concerned with a mode of consciousness that has to do with the way objects relate to one another. It deals with images and patterns, it recognises musical rhythms and melodies. It is probably the source of intuitive insights and imagination. Those individuals who have a well-developed right mode of consciousness are usually seen as 'artistic' or gifted. Our educational system tends to damp down this mode of consciousness and rewards more left-sided activities, like reasoning and reading and mathematical ability. The way our society is ordered illustrates how we select and reinforce these left-sided activities. When faced with a difficulty or problem, we tend immediately to 'think' our way out of it. Yet some of the most creative solutions and ideas arrive when our right side is given free reign.

Exercise IV
Allow any tune to come into your mind. Start humming the tune – what feelings or sensations arise in you as you hum this tune? How much can you learn about your true inner feelings by observing which tune arises spontaneously? Is it a happy tune or a sad tune, is it a tune associated with someone in particular or a specific event in your life? You can use this simple exercise from time to time to check out your inner feelings or recapture a lost memory of importance.

Exercise V

Draw a tree. On a large piece of paper draw a tree using coloured crayons or pencils. Draw any tree that comes into your mind, do not think about it too much. Draw the tree in the ground and any objects that might be around it. Draw the sky and the landscape. Are there other trees by it or is it on its own? When you have finished drawing the tree, hold the picture up, possibly to a friend or, if you are on your own, to yourself and then describe the tree. As you describe the tree, instead of saying, 'This tree is . . .', use the first person singular and say, 'I am a holly tree and I am . . . etc., etc.'. After finishing this exercise, reflect on what this tells you about yourself. How accurate were you? In what ways was the tree a drawing of yourself? Repeat this exercise from time to time, keeping your trees, and observe how they change and how they reflect, or not, your own development.

Exercise VI – Visualisation

Visualisation is a way of using the 'mind's eye' to obtain information about yourself or your situation. It can also be used to produce physical changes within the body and help you to relax. Allowing yourself to hold on to an image of peacefulness can help to bring about that state often more effectively than willing yourself to be peaceful – 'I must be peaceful'. Visualisation, or the use of imagery, has developed into a major clinical tool for many mental as well as physical disorders. Consciously constructed images (called either active imagination, guided fantasies or directed day-dreaming) have been used to treat patients with asthma, heart attack and cancer. Simonton, who pioneered this method for cancer patients, encouraged them to imagine the cancer cells being bombarded by antibodies. He would ask his patients actually to draw the cancer cells and then hold on to the image of them being destroyed. His initial results have been encouraging and many more clinicians are now experimenting with this approach. You can use visualisation to aid your ability to work with your breathing, relaxation and meditation. On other occasions you can use this technique to reduce pain or explore creatively a problem or difficulty you are currently experiencing.

Visualisation with breathing

Lie down on the floor or bed and follow the instructions for diaphragmatic breathing. When your breathing is quiet and rhythmical, imagine a circle in front of your eyes. As you breathe in, imagine you are drawing half a circle with your breath. As you breathe out, imagine your breath completing the circle. Repeat this a few times, trying to make the circle as smooth and round as you can. After a few minutes allow this image to go and imagine you are breathing in from the tips of your toes to the top of your skull and as you breathe out you breathe out from the top of your skull to the tips of your toes. Try and imagine the breath actually travelling all the way up and down the spine.

Visualisation and relaxation

Once you have achieved a state of progressive relaxation as described on p. 36, allow a picture of a favourite, restful place to develop in front of your closed eyes. It might be a mountainside, or by the sea, or a special room. Allow whatever image occurs to form and develop the picture slowly by filling in the various objects or items associated with it. Look at each object in turn and heighten the colours associated with the object. Now fill the atmosphere a little more with the sounds and smells associated with this place. If your attention wanders, gently bring it back to the image and allow the picture to reform. After 5–10 minutes, gradually let go of the image and bring your attention slowly back to your body and then slowly back to the room you are in.

Visualisation and meditation

In the last section, we described a meditation exercise using a sound as a focus for the mind. You can practise a similar exercise using a real picture or a created image. We do this spontaneously when looking into a fire or watching something on the distant horizon. The yogis developed special pictures to look at during meditation called mandalas, which were usually circular patterned images. You can use a picture of a respected mentor or sage (orthodox Christians used icons) or if you meditate with your eyes closed, you can create an image of a face or candle or clock face.

Visualisation for pain relief

It is usually necessary to have acquired some expertise for this process to be effective in severe pain. First, use your breath to reduce the tension surrounding the painful part. Close your eyes, focus on your breathing as described previously, slow your breathing down, then imagine that you are breathing in and out through the painful part – joint, tooth, head. As you breathe into the part, imagine a warm glow being carried into the part by your breath, and as you breathe out, imagine the pain and tension being carried away by the breath. An additional image that helps some people is to imagine a dial which they can turn up or down – turning the dial one way decreases the pain, and turning the dial the other increases the pain.

Visualisation for creative exploration

Find a comfortable position where you will be undisturbed for 10–15 minutes. Either sit in a comfortable position or lie down on the floor or bed. Close your eyes and begin to breathe slowly and rhythmically. Go through a relaxation routine as before.

Now imagine that you are a rose-bush – picture the rose-bush in front of you. What colour are the roses, how many of them are there, is the rose-bush on its own, what kind of rose-bush are you, where are you growing, what are your roots like, what is the soil like, what are the stems like, what are the thorns like, how does it feel to be a rose-bush, what is your life like as a rose-bush? Allow your imagination free rein and follow it willingly.

After a few minutes, let the image go, become aware of your body and then the room, and finally open your eyes.

Try and recapture what you have found out about yourself either by writing it down, drawing it or telling a friend.

Working with feelings

Our feelings are often the most individual part of ourselves, and usually the most difficult to manage. Feelings are a mixture of both a mental and physical experience. Observable physical changes occur when someone is overwhelmed with a feeling, such as anger, sadness, joy. We look at people's faces or posture and are able to detect how they are feeling. We get some guidance at school about our bodies and minds but very rarely are we given any advice as to how to manage our feelings. More often than not we are told in many different ways 'not to show our feelings'. Even to talk about managing feelings seems inappropriate. Yet there are occasions when we need to moderate our feelings or when the phy ical experience is so distressing that it is necessary to find ways of reducing the discomfort. Not all feelings are negative, and the joy, happiness and sheer ecstasy enjoyed in pursuing pleasurable pursuits are as important as the sadness, misery and unhappiness that are part of most people's human experience. Feelings are neither 'bad' nor 'good', they are there, to be experienced. Nevertheless a long-held feeling of resentment or guilt or anger may well produce a chronic mental attitude of physical difficulty. Norman Cousins, in his book *Anatomy of an Illness*, describes how a positive feeling of happiness and laughter can moderate illness and reverse symptoms.

Exercise VII – Increasing awareness
Below is a list of emotions (feelings that most of us have experienced from time to time). Mark those that you are aware of having and indicate how often you 'show' your feelings.

Exercise VIII – Recapturing a feeling
Write of a feeling you would like to find out more about. Try and remember when you last felt angry or frightened. Notice what physical sensations occur in your body. Where do you tense – does your face change – is your breathing different? Now notice what thoughts arise as you remember that feeling. You may choose to accentuate the feeling and the physical changes to increase your awareness for a minute. This exercise will help make you more familiar with the way your body/mind responds to feelings.

Exercise IX – Understanding your feelings
Complete the following sentences:
  – I feel angry when ....
  – I feel that my anger is ....
  – When others express their anger towards me I feel ....
  ....
  – I feel that the anger of others is ....
You can repeat this exercise with other feelings that may give you difficulty.

121

FEELING	EXPERIENCED				REVEALED (SHOWN)			
	1 Never	2 Rarely	3 Some- times	4 Often	1 Never	2 Rarely	3 Some- times	4 Often
ANGER								
IRRITATION								
FRUSTRATION								
RESENTMENT								
GUILT								
SADNESS								
LONELINESS								
UNHAPPINESS								
DEPRESSION								
ANXIETY								
FEAR								
PANIC								
SURPRISE								
EXCITEMENT								
ELATION								
JOY								
HAPPINESS								
SATISFACTION								
SYMPATHY								
JEALOUSY								
ENVY								
BOREDOM								

Exercise X – Moving thoughts to help with feelings

Feelings almost invariably either follow a thought or are preceded by a thought. Thinking your way into a depression or a state of fear is not uncommon, and it is therefore possible to reverse the process and 'think' yourself out of a distressful feeling. All too often the individual is caught up by the physical nature of the feeling and is unable to 'think'. The previous exercise will help as it may reveal the irrational nature of the thoughts. It is necessary on occasions to use the breathing exercises to provide you with a 'breathing space' so that you can allow thoughts to develop. Often our feelings operate on a two-point scale – either we have none or the emotion is so intense that it is overwhelming. Whilst in a calm and balanced state, it can be helpful to let the alternate emotional responses that could be more appropriate in the situation you are faced with emerge. Much of *assertiveness* training is concerned with separating inappropriate agression (rage, fury) from assertive statements ('Please do not do that again'). Panic or severe anxiety about a piece of work can be altered to concern. Guilt at having caused someone some pain can be modified to regret and apology.

Exercise XI – Letting go of your feelings

Much of psychotherapy and the confessional for that matter is concerned with giving people the space to 'get something off their chest'. Most of us have had experiences where the emotional impact of that experience has not been sufficiently well dealt with. It might be that we repressed a feeling (anger at losing a job, sadness at the break-up of a marriage) or that our feelings were not accepted as valid by our family or friends. Repressed and unexpressed emotions cause havoc with our mental line and subsequent relationships. Arriving home after a frustrating day at work, feeling resentful, irritable and angry, is a recipe for disaster on the home front. Discharging such feelings is as important as being aware of the need to cry and sob and weep when something distressing has occurred (a bereavement or a disappointment).

Anger and frustration can often be helped by physical effort – running or jogging, or hitting a tennis racquet, or a mattress or pillow. Shouting at the top of your voice in your car as you drive home or in a park may appear odd and unusual, but it is much better than shouting at your wife/husband or children. Letting go of tears is more difficult and it may require the help of a friend, counsellor or sympathetic doctor. Tears contain a raised level of the stress hormone *cortisol* and they are the natural way of relieving the body and mind of stress.

Working with irrational thoughts

Statements such as 'it's all in the mind', 'mind over matter', 'positive thinking' illustrate the belief that we can train our minds to think in a particular way which will then produce changes both in our feelings and in our attitudes and relationships. There is no doubt that this sort of activity is possible, but the danger is that if it is pursued to its extreme, the idea that sadness or regret or dislike or even hate is only a 'negative emotion or thought' develops. A holistic approach involves accepting both positive and negative aspects of ourselves and not necessarily denying or repressing the negative. With that word of caution 'positive thinking' can be of great help for people who habitually put themselves down or feel worthless and hopeless. Giving yourself a few phrases to repeat in a difficult or stressful situation can help you to cope with that situation, e.g.:

Preparation	'There's nothing to worry about'
	'I'm going to be all right'
	'It's easier once you get started'
Confronting	'Take it step by step'
	'I can only do my best'
	'I can get help if I need it'
Coping with fear	'Relax *now*'
	'Breathe deeply'
	'There is an end to it'
Reinforcing success	'I did it'
	'Next time I won't worry so much'
	'I am able to relax away anxiety'

Learning from dreams

Freud said that dreams were 'the royal road to the unconscious' – by which he meant that they contained information about our past, and some now believe our future, which is not normally accessible to us during the waking state. We all dream regularly, although few of us remember our dreams. Many manuals both popular and serious are available to describe what your dreams tell you about yourself. People pay large sums of money to go to psychoanalysts for years to uncover their hidden meaning. Unfortunately, one of the major misunderstandings that people have about dreams is that they have to be 'analysed' or 'understood'. Of more importance is that the images and memories recreated by the dream are experienced, either directly or indirectly, by writing about the dream, or drawing it, or making a plasticine model of some of the figures present. Keeping a dream journal is a helpful beginning, but don't feel you have to rush away and find out what your dreams mean. If you remember a dream, write it down and then during a relaxation or a meditation or a jog, or in the bath, allow the images of the dream to resurface and using the guided fantasy technique (Chapter 6), build on the images of your dreams and follow the developments without interfering too much with your thoughts. Jung felt the greatest problem for the western mind was that it needed to be freed from the cramp of conscious control. Dreams are the mind's way of allowing that to happen. More important than what they mean is that you should experience their impact.

8

SEX AND SEXUALITY

Even though in the last twenty or thirty years there appears to have been a revolution in our attitude towards sex, for many this is still a troubled aspect of their life. Indeed it could be said that it is because the sexual act has become so explicit and books, magazines, articles, films and television programmes on the subject are now so freely available that the problems of ignorance have been replaced with the problems of 'performance anxiety'. The sexual act has lost its meaning and has been replaced with the search for the multiple orgasm or the 'zipless fuck'. Knowledge about the physical nature of our bodies is obviously necessary to enjoy the act of making love.

Our sexuality, however, is more than just a physical expression. At the deepest level of making love it is a physical, emotional and spiritual act. In that sense it is truly an integration of body, mind and spirit, but we can help someone else achieve it as well. In this final act the blending of two human beings with a capacity to receive love and give love is, as one psychiatrist put it, 'an interpenetrating harmonious mix up'. We all yearn to be held, contain and love someone else. In the act of making love, we are given that opportunity to make peace with ourselves and another human being. We do not have to be athletic performers or achieve the heights of physical ecstasy. For many, simply holding hands, gently massaging, cuddling, comforting, hugging with full awareness and a positive intention to love and be loved is more than sufficient. The important aspect seems to be the willingness to 'let go' and surrender oneself for a few minutes in the company of someone else. Truly to 'be there' for some other human being is more important than getting the position right and having the perfect technique or latest sexual aid.

127

Like everything else we have said before, understanding your sexuality starts with awareness. Make a list of all the reasons why you make love. Be honest with yourself. Is it because of heightened sexual desire, or habit? Is it because you don't want to say no or because you like giving your partner pleasure? Is it because you are lonely, miserable and unhappy or because you are angry, fed up and tense? It probably is a mixture of all these reasons and many more. The difficulties and problems that arise in the sexual act have many origins and, as we have already said, it is not essential to reach the peak of physical ecstasy to achieve the state of union with another human being. It is necessary though to have some understanding of your needs, physical as well as emotional, to help you towards that state of union.

Sex and your body

Take a good look at your body and increase your awareness of those essentially sexual parts of you. This chapter is not going to include the kind of detail you obtain from many of the excellent books on the market and some readers might find it helpful to obtain some of these manuals listed at the end of the book.

For *men* the penis is the primary sexual organ and in its flaccid state will vary in size and shape. During puberty the penis starts growing and the testes in the scrotum enlarge and produce increased male hormone (testosterone) as well as sperms. The pubic hair coarsens and the prostate gland increases its secretions. Both before puberty and after, the penis undergoes spontaneous erection. This can often be worrisome for parents as well as guilt-making for boys. Spontaneous erections continue to occur throughout adult life and are normal accompaniments of dreams and sleep. The penis achieves a size of between 6 and 7 inches during erection and although much has been written about sexual potency and size, most of it is fanciful and unhelpful. Masturbation is an almost universal act amongst young boys and adolescents and some adult males can well continue to draw benefit or pleasure from masturbation both within a loving relationship as well as in situations where there is no other partner. Many men have their foreskin removed during circumcision and this will help prevent minor infections, help with hygiene and for some will prolong their ability to maintain an erection during intercourse. The thin piece of tissue between the tip of the penis and the base of the glans called the *fraenulum* is a particularly sensitive sexual area for the male. Other sexually sensitive areas for men include the nipples, mouth and tongue, inner area of thighs, the anus and surrounding skin, the ear-lobes and soles of the feet.

In fact it is true to say that almost any part of the body can derive sexual pleasure and that the excitement of sharing and discovering forms part of the mystery of sex. Men derive pleasure not only through the direct stimulation of sexual organs but through sound, sight and smell, as shown by the ever popular expositions of female nudity in advertisements, books and films. Men can increase their sexual arousal by ensuring that those senses of sound, sight and smell receive equal stimulation during love-making. Semen is made up of sperms (produced by the testes and stored in the epididymes). These travel along the vas deferens and are added to by secretions from the prostate gland and cowpers gland. The amount of semen produced varies according to continence and frequency of love-making and the quantity of the ejaculate is only minimally affected by sterilisation.

Men are most sexually potent during adolescence and their early twenties. Sexual athleticism can continue well into the seventies and eighties but for the most part, men find that less frequent sexual activity is perfectly acceptable. Older men are able to maintain an erection for longer and thus prolong the pleasure both they and their partners derive.

Male Sexuality

It is interesting to note that though there has been an intense interest in the nature of female sexuality, little has been written about the basis of male sexuality. It is taken for granted by many that the man is the active partner in a heterosexual couple initiating sex, determining its frequency and taking command over its performance. In other words, male sexuality has been linked to power, aggression, drive and control. For many men, the sexual act is an act involving the domination and submission of women. It has often been used for that very fact. Rape, forced sex, sadistic practices, promiscuity, prostitution are, in part, symptoms of the male's aggressive drive being linked to his sex drive. Many women are no longer willing to accept this link from their menfolk, and for sensitive men the next twenty, thirty years will prove to be a difficult and confusing time as they learn to unlearn the link between sexuality and aggression.

The issue is not that power, force, drive and determination are necessarily inappropriate during love-making but that the sexual act for men should not be a substitute for their inadequacies in these areas. If a woman is continually used to appease the man's feeling of inadequacy, then she is being used and the relationship between the man and the woman runs the risk of becoming stagnant. The resolution of this dilemma, as so often in this book, is found in the awareness surrounding the act of love-making. If a man has his sense of worth restored by making active, forceful love to a woman who is receptive and understanding of his needs, then both will be enriched. If, however, a woman is subjugated and coerced into a submissive role by an insensitive and unappreciative male, then both will have been diminished. Men will have to learn other ways of expressing their sexuality. Receiving and giving pleasure with tenderness and gentleness, surrendering and letting go of one's own immediate need for gratification, require men to alter their accepted view of their sexuality. The man is often caught up with frequency of sex, and achieving an orgasm at all costs. The journey is more important than the place of arrival. Exploring the nature of one's sexuality is a way of exploring one's personality. Finding a partner who will join you in the journey and act as a partner, guide, teacher and pupil at different moments is for many the highest achievement that can be attained in their lives.

Homosexuality

The increasing tolerance towards gay men and women has been welcomed by many in our society. With it has come the exploration of the homosexual nature of all men and women which for many is still difficult and dangerous. It is helpful to differentiate between *gender* and 'sex'. Gender refers to the traditional male and female attributes: *male* signifies active, penetrating, outgoing, goal-oriented; and *female* signifies receptive, nuturing, giving, process-oriented. Sex refers both to the sexual organs we are born with and to the sexual preference (homosexual, heterosexual) we have. A useful diagram to illustrate this will give you an opportunity to become aware of your own sexuality and the balance of *sex* and *gender* present in your own make-up.

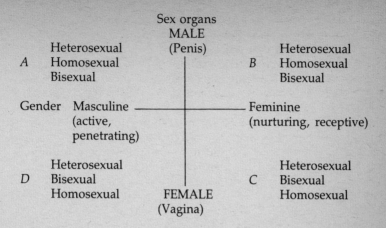

From the chart, it is possible to work out twelve different group-ings. Human observation suggests that although the majority of us keep closely within one group, for many the exploration of the different groups is an increasing development of under-standing our sexuality.

A1 *Sex organ* – Penis *Gender* – Masculine *Sexual preference* – female
At its worst this is the stereotyped image of the aggressive rampant sexual male animal devouring and raping the submissive woman. At its best, it is the predominant nature of most men in our culture today.

A2 *Sex organ* – Penis *Gender* – Masculine *Sexual preference* – Male
The active assertive male homosexual is an increasing feature of our culture and the recent exposition of Holly-wood idols as homosexual is an illustration of how preva-lent this grouping has become.

A3 *Sex organ* – Penis *Gender* – Masculine *Sexual preference* – Bisexual
In many cultures, especially in the Middle East, this is a not uncommon cluster and considered quite normal. Many 'normal' men will explore homosexual expression of their sexuality during adolescence and early adulthood but return to a predominant heterosexual expression.

131

B1 *Sex organ* – Penis *Gender* – Female *Sexual preference* – Female
This is a sensitive, gentle, nurturing man who loves and respects his female partner. She may at times find him too passive and not sufficiently dominating. However, for many liberated women, this may be the ideal mate. For men, attempting to achieve the sensitivity and receptivity required to carry out this role is the challenge they are most likely to face in our current society.

B2 *Sex organ* – Penis *Gender* – Female *Sexual preference* – Male
The stereotyped passive homosexual is the classical description of this mode – such adjectives as 'queen', 'gay', 'queer' are normally used to describe in a pejorative way how society views this sort of behaviour. Nevertheless, increasing numbers of men are enjoying dressing up, wearing make-up and jewellery. They are discovering the pleasure of expressing their sexuality in more feminine ways – without necessarily expressing their sexuality in a homosexual manner.

B3 *Sex organ* – Penis *Gender* – Female *Sexual preference* – Bisexual
This is a natural development for many men from the previous role and can be found amongst many of our pop stars and theatre personalities.

C1 *Sex organ* – Vagina *Gender* – Feminine *Sexual preference* – Male
The predominant role for many women who live as wives and mothers supporting and looking after their active husbands and sons. During sex they adopt a more passive role but can be and often are an essential factor in preserving family life as we know it. For increasing numbers of women this has become an unsatisfactory role and the impact of the women's movement has been to give women an opportunity to question whether they really want to live out their lives expressing themselves solely in this mode.

C2 *Sex organ* – Vagina *Gender* – Feminine *Sexual preference* – Female
The passive partner in a lesbian relationship – many young girls pass through this phase and develop crushes on teachers or older schoolgirls.

C3 *Sex organ* – Vagina *Gender* – Feminine *Sexual preference* – Bisexual

Many women who have unsatisfactory sex lives living in a marriage have found a fulfilment and acceptance in a lesbian relationship they never thought possible. The general increase in lesbian expression of sexual love is a result amongst other factors of the inability of men to recognise the nature of 'feminine sexuality', in their own make-up as well as that of their partner.

D1 *Sex organ* – Vagina *Gender* – Masculine *Sexual preference* – Male

At its worst, this is the aggressive, demanding, devouring woman who takes command and expresses her sexuality directly and without fear. At best this can be the liberated woman who knows what she wants and makes sure she gets it, if necessary by teaching her mate how to give it to her. Many men have difficulty in relating to this sort of woman, who is an increasing feature of our culture. Men experience difficulty in maintaining their image of themselves as the 'potent partner' and the increasing incidence of impotence is a result of the challenge this sort of woman places on her male partner.

D2 *Sex organ* – Vagina *Gender* – Masculine *Sexual preference* – Female

The classic 'butch' in a lesbian relationship, and a stage many women go through in exploring their own liberated sexuality.

D3 *Sex organ* – Vagina *Gender* – Masculine *Sexual preference* – Bisexual

Unlike the male bisexual, this role is not as common, but with the increasing exploration of the nature of sexuality it will no doubt be an increasing development.

It is important to underline that it is not necessary to express one's sexuality in an 'active way' but it does help to understand and increase one's awareness. Understanding the focus of your sexual needs and drives can allow you to overcome the difficulties you may encounter as well as increase your ability to be of help to your partner.

The female body

The vulva includes the vaginal lips (labia), the clitoris and the vagina proper. The clitoris is the most sensitive sexual organ in the woman and the area from which most physical pleasure is derived. Orgasm is most often achieved through clitoral stimulation, and the willingness on the part of both partners to explore this part of the female anatomy during foreplay is one of the necessary 'techniques' in love-making. The vagina contains two glands opening just on the inside wall. These glands are thought to secrete lubricant which allows for easy penetration during intercourse. Like men, women have additional sexual anatomical zones which include the breasts and nipples, the mouth, tongue and lips, the neck and ear lobes as well as the thighs, anus and feet. Recently the area of the perineum (between anus and vagina) has been found to contain a large collection of nerve endings which are particularly sexually sensitive. This so-called 'G' spot has no doubt been located by many couples well before the anatomists and sexologists described it.

The ovaries which secrete the eggs and the female hormone oestrogen are found inside the female pelvis and are suspended over the fallopian tubes which carry the eggs into the wings of the uterus (womb). The cervix is that portion of the womb which protrudes into the vagina and can be felt by most women by placing two fingers into the vagina whilst squatting. It is unusual for the penis to be long enough to reach the cervix during intercourse but on occasions this can occur. The skin is probably the largest sexual organ in the body and it is important to be aware of how much pleasure can be obtained through touching, hugging, stroking, massaging. The influence of menstruation on both the sexual organs and the sexual desire is an additional factor for women that is not too well understood by women, let alone men.

Development of secondary sexual characteristics starts earlier in girls than boys but is not usually accompanied with an increase in sexual desire. The first few years of menstruation may be anovulatory, i.e. eggs are not released. Masturbation, although not uncommon amongst girls, is not as universal as it is in boys and the nature of sexual arousal in girls manifests itself in different ways. During adulthood women do become aware of times of increased sexual arousal akin to 'heat' in other animals. This varies with different cultures and different women, although it is generally found to coincide with ovulation in mid-cycle. The freedom from childbearing that effective contraception has produced has made it possible for many more women to take a more active role in determining when or when not to have intercourse. The female of the human species is one of the few species that is sexually receptive throughout her reproductive phase. This does and can continue following the cessation of periods and the onset of menopause. Many of the changes occurring during the menopause need not have any effect on sexual drive and interest. For many women this can become a time of renewed sexual activity. Changes in breast tissue, skin and volva occurring as part of the normal aging process do not inhibit the sexuality of women.

Sexual union

For many men and women an active, enjoyable sexual life can be the source of great comfort and joy. Difficulties in sexual expression can bring distress, pain and depression. Love-making is at one and the same time both a simple natural expression of being human and a complex physical and psychological obstacle course. We are not attempting to provide a sexual manual but will mention aspects that are important to a more holistic attitude. The bringing together of two naked human bodies in a warm and private atmosphere is often the first hurdle to overcome. Being aware of the room and the bed, allowing for changes and introducing new sounds (music) or smells (incense, perfume) will help to increase the sensual nature of love-making. Finding out what you want and like and taking responsibility for obtaining it will follow from your own increased awareness. Similarly, finding out about your partner's needs and wants is part of the process of learning about your mate.

As has been mentioned before, the skin is probably the most underused and neglected organ of our bodies. The need for closeness and union can more often be expressed through touching and hugging than through intercourse. Learning how to do simple massage both on yourself and your partner will enhance your ability to give as well as receive. Obtain some massage oil and start today. Stroking, rubbing, cupping, gentling, kneading, are skills that each human adult should know more about. Much of the healing that comes from such diverse traditions as osteopathy, acupressure, shiatsu, reflexology, chiropractice, physiotherapy, are the direct results of the increased touching that forms part of these therapies. For many years the 'laying on of hands' was an integral part of healing for all good doctors. It is now too often neglected and even frowned on. Spending time to touch and be touched before actual intercourse will enhance the quality and depth of the union that is possible. Women need to teach men as well as themselves how and where they want to be touched. Clitoral stimulation is more than just a vigorous 'scrubbing brush' activity.

The more adventurous sexual couples will explore the use of the mouth and tongue, but underlying all the 'foreplay' is the willingness to receive as well as to give. Many couples will work out a pattern of mutuality when they take it in turn. Simultaneous orgasm is a fantasy of the film-makers and, although occurring on occasions, is the exception rather than the rule. Actual intercourse need not be the final act on every occasion. Helping the partner to masturbate or sharing a mutual masturbation may be a particularly intimate form of expressing one's concern and love. During times of illness or pregnancy many couples will find themselves experimenting with other ways of achieving sexual release and satisfaction. For those of you temporarily separated from your partner or not in a relationship, many will find that masturbation can be an important part in retaining physical balance. At times of increased stress and tension, some find that masturbation can be a perfectly appropriate way to relax.

Penetration and positions

Change and experimentation is perfectly appropriate in sexual intercourse, but you should not worry if you have arrived at a comfortable and acceptable position and do not feel the need for a change. The various athletic positions found in sexual manuals are there to be used if there is a shared interest. More important is allowing for a change in roles: who initiates sexual activity, who takes the lead, are you able to follow as well as lead? During intercourse itself, experiment with your body – men can learn to be receptive and follow whilst women can learn to take command. The depth of union can be increased by relaxing during intercourse keeping the eyes open and looking into your partner's eyes. Developing the ability to make intercourse a more meditative process will allow couples to experience a sense of bliss and peace which is of a different quality from that achieved by vigorous active intercourse. Lying in your partner's arms without moving whilst the erect penis is in the vagina will increase both the physical as well as the psychological experience.

The nature of the female orgasm has been well researched and written about in recent years and Masters and Johnson have helped many doctors and sexologists understand how to guide women through the difficulties they may experience in achieving orgasm. Feminists and psychoanalysts have long debated over the site of orgasm – whether it is clitoral or vaginal – but it is now apparent both from the scientific studies as well as from women's own experience that not only can they and do they achieve multiple orgasm through clitoral stimulation but that for many women a vaginal orgasm is a different but equally satisfactory method of achieving pleasure during intercourse.

Difficulties, problems and hang-ups

Male
If impotence (failure to produce an erection) persists, it is important to obtain a medical opinion as some reversible medical conditions can cause this problem. Certain drugs, alcohol and general fatigue are not infrequent factors and most men will have experienced occasions when an erection fails to materialise. The attendant anxiety can often produce a vicious circle and fear of impotence in itself will cause impotence. There is a gradual increase in the incidence of impotence with age, although many elderly men continue to have satisfactory sexual activity well into their seventies and eighties. Impotence can be helped by a loving and gentle partner and the answer is often found by focussing on the non-sexual aspects of love-making – holding, touching, comforting and decreasing the tension by doing the relaxation exercises described earlier. Where fatigue and low sexual drive are factors, remember that pleasure and satisfaction do not require sexual penetration. Nevertheless, manual or oral stimulation of the penis will help many men achieve an erection.

Premature ejaculation is more common than impotence and can cause much distress and embarrassment. Sexologists define premature ejaculation as the failure to maintain an erection sufficient to satisfy the female partner on more than 50% of occasions. More frequent intercourse can often help to solve this problem, as can the sensate focussing and squeeze technique as described by Masters and Johnson. The latter is easy to perform, given co-operation, and is mostly successful. The man achieves an erection and before he reaches ejaculation his partner squeezes the head of the penis moderately hard for 3–4 seconds. The man usually loses his erection and the procedure is repeated a few times. The penis is then inserted in the vagina and again when the man feels he is nearing ejaculation he withdraws and the squeeze is reapplied.

Special problems such as pain on intercourse or more lasting impotence will require specialised help. More complex situations involving promiscuity or sado-masochism are beyond the scope of this book, but it is important to mention that many of the so-called sexual perversions are perfectly normal and as long as no one is harmed and both partners are acquiescent, indulging in one's sexual fantasies is a perfectly acceptable form of adult play. Indeed, the sexual bedchamber can be seen as the playpen for adults. Like playpens, it needs to be safe and the toys used need to be non-toxic, not dangerous and not too complicated. You will find like a child that you have your favourite game but that the occasional new game will increase your interest and help you explore your strengths as well as your limitations.

Female
Painful intercourse may be the result of poor lubrication or vaginismus (spasm of the pelvic muscles). Other causes include infections or vaginal skin problems and occasional pelvic infections. Lack of lubrication can be easy to overcome by using external lubrication (the best form is saliva), but a dry vagina suggests that one partner is not sufficiently attentive to the other partner's needs. Vaginismus results from more complex sexual difficulties which may have to do with difficulties in the relationship – if the female partner is unwilling or has little desire for intercourse, forcing a penis inside her will not help. Again, it is important to stress that sexual penetration is not the be all and end all of sexual communion. Women who persistently fail to achieve orgasm may be quite happy about this even though their male partners may not. However, the gentle exploration and stimulation of the vagina and vulva together with guided touching of the clitoral area will help some women achieve orgasm.

Relaxing and reducing the element of performance is an important accompaniment of any attempt to help with sexual problems. Once the woman is sufficiently aroused, experimenting with positions will help to increase the potential for orgasm – side to side can be more conducive in achieving female orgasm. The penis can be left inside the vagina and the slower rate that women take to achieve orgasm needs to be recognised. Allowing the woman to determine the frequency of thrusting movement will give her more control. Finally, both oral stimulation of the clitoris and the use of a vibrator can be helpful. More often than not it is helping the woman explore her own sexual anatomy using her fingers and encouraging her to masturbate that will allow her to achieve orgasm. Once orgasm is achieved, it is easier to reach orgasm again in the future.

9

RELATION-SHIPS

'Create spaces in your togetherness' – Gibran

Well, at last – we've arrived at the really difficult area. For there is no doubt that of all our human activities, relating to our fellow human beings appears to give us most problems. For some, especially the elderly and bereaved, the difficulty is not having any relationships at all. For parents, the difficulty is with children, especially during adolescence – worrying about different standards and values, feeling unappreciated and used by children who keep their rooms resembling a tip, wear outrageous clothes, play loud music and, more seriously, experiment with drugs. For children, the difficulty may be having parents who are constantly quarrelling, or possibly not having a father or mother at all. The breakdown in relationships between husbands and wives keeps our courts busy with an ever-increasing divorce rate (1 in 3 marriages end in divorce, as do 1 in 2 second marriages). For some, the problem lies in relationships at work – a boss who is tyrannical or unsympathetic, other fellow workers who are rejecting or simply unfriendly. Competitiveness in business, professional and academic life is notorious for producing a 'rat-race' attitude that makes the work environment positively harmful.

The problems between individual people can be magnified into problems between groups, and we read daily of attacks on ethnic minorities or the warring groups in Northern Ireland (Protestant v. Catholic), India (Hindu v. Sikh v. Muslim), South Africa (White v. Black). The history of mankind is in part the history of misunderstandings, miscommunications and broken relationships between individuals, groups and nations. And yet we are a gregarious animal. Our instinct is to pair and mate, form groups, create

141

societies. A happy and mutually satisfying marriage can be the greatest achievement for any human being. Our ability to think evil of our fellow, plan and plot destruction, maim and torture helpless victims, is balanced by our ability to show concern and compassion, to sacrifice and restore, to love and hold. Is it a fruitless dream to hope for a family, society or nation where the inequalities and injustices of our relationships are for ever eradicated?

We can only, as in the other chapters, provide a brief outline of some of the processes that occur in relationships and indicate ways in which improving communications between people and within groups can sometimes be achieved. Progress in this area of our life is painfully slow, but if we are to make use of all the breathing, relaxation, meditation and diet work we have outlined, surely it is to enable us to improve the quality of our human relationships.

Projection – or which way is your finger pointing?

Projection is a term used in psychoanalysis, but as a concept it is as old as mankind. The Bible says, 'Thou hypocrite, cast out first the beam out of thine own eye; and then shalt thou see clearly to cast out the mote out of thy brother's eye' (Matthew 7:5). Thomas à Kempis wrote: 'What a man is inwardly that he will see outwardly.' Projection is the process by which we first 'repress' and then cast out those aspects of ourselves which we do not like or do not accept. Someone who sees himself as 'good' will see 'evil' around him – he will repress his own negative thoughts of envy or lust or greed and will 'project' them on to other people. When he points a finger at them, one finger, usually the index, will be directed towards the other person. *He is bad* – but three fingers will be pointing directly towards himself. Projection is a necessary part of the way we relate to our external world. We project not only those negative aspects of ourselves but also the positive ones. If we do not believe we possess charm or poise or beauty or goodness within ourselves, we project, like a film projector, these qualities on to other people – film stars, politicians, religious leaders.

Jung went so far as to say that 'everyone creates for himself a series of more or less imaginary relationships based essentially on projection'. Jung felt we all have a very basic instinct (like hunger or sex) for becoming whole people. This means that we need to reclaim those projected bits of ourselves and accept them as ours. In our relationships, we therefore seek out those individuals who carry those qualities we admire most but also dislike most. In marriage one may find that after a while husband and wife come to dislike those very qualities that first attracted them to their spouse. The policeman who upholds law and order spends his life chasing the criminal, who represents the projected part of the policeman – the tendency to break laws and disturb order. The husband who sees himself as rational, intellectual and clear may quarrel incessantly with his wife whom he sees as irrational, emotional and scatty. The polarities – good–bad; emotional–intellectual; strong–weak – are drawn to each other and if one or other person in the relationship does not accept that they are 'projecting' the opposite quality, then sparks fly.

At times, relationships will form between like and like – and then the couple or group will project the unwanted quality outside their circle. We thus see how the 'them and us' situation arises and the terrible consequences that occur when this process is magnified to states and nations. The Nazis 'projected' all their unwanted qualities on the Jews. The frequency of wars and tribal conflicts is often a reflection on how much 'projection' is taking place – the enemy need not always be *bad* but he invariably becomes so if the conflict persists. Being aware *that* we project and learning how to withdraw these projections will go some way to help creating more stable relationships.

The person behind the mask

The process of projection necessitates our having to wear a 'mask'. Most of us are aware to a greater or lesser extent of how this 'mask' helps us deal with our external world. Part of our education by both our parents and schools is learning how to curb our need for immediate satisfaction. We are taught how to smile and say please and thank you even if we do not feel like it. We are cautioned against showing our negative feelings and we arrive in adulthood more or less 'socialised' in a certain pattern of behaviour acceptable to the society we live in. In the meantime our true feelings and thoughts about situations and experiences which we have had accumulate unexpressed and often unnoticed even by us. We learn to adapt and conform, we learn to 'relate' to our fellow human beings by hiding our true feelings. Now obviously some of this process is perfectly appropriate. Unfortunately, often the mask we put on becomes the real person, but this mask is held on by external artefacts like wigs or make-up or clothes, although the opposite may also be true – the artefacts may be revealing more about the person behind the mask than they are hiding. Even more complicating is the fact that not only may there be many different masks but there may be many different people behind the mask. It is no surprise therefore that communications between people are so fraught with misunderstanding and usually end up in knots, as has been so well documented by R. D. Laing in his book *Knots*. An example of both projection and masks is the following poem:

Jack is afraid of Jill
Jill is afraid of Jack
Jack is more afraid of Jill
If Jack thinks
that Jill thinks
that Jack is afraid of Jill
Since Jack is afraid
that Jill will think that
Jack is afraid

Jack is not afraid of Jill

So that Jill will be more afraid of Jack

and since Jill is afraid
that Jack will think that
Jill is afraid
Jill pretends that
Jill is not afraid of Jack

Thus
Jack tries to make Jill afraid by not being afraid of Jill
and Jill tries to make Jack afraid
by not being afraid of Jack

Fortunately not all our relationships or communications get into quite this tangled mess, but given the complexity of our abilities, it is amazing that we get it right so often.

One helpful way to begin to disentangle some of these knots is to examine both your 'inner person' and then your 'mask'. You may need help from friends and colleagues to find out how your mask is seen, but let's start with the inner person. A useful scheme is provided by transactional analysis – a form of psychotherapy that was developed by Dr Eric Berne. He identified three types of inner personalities or ego states that most of us possess and from which most of us communicate. He called these ego states *Parent*, *Adult* and *Child*.

Parent

The parent part of the inner personality is the part that hands out the shoulds, oughts and musts. It is the judging and critical part of ourselves and keeps a record of all the dos and don'ts in our life. It can also be the nurturing and protective part of our personality. It looks after us in times of trouble or distress and keeps a kindly eye out for any difficulties. The parent part of us is influenced by our own real parents, teachers, people in authority that we come across during the early part of our life. Much as we may have been encouraged or supported by our real parents, so our own 'inner parent' may provide us with those attributes that we can call upon or share with others.

Whether your inner parent is more critical and blaming or supportive and encouraging will in part depend on the sort of parenting you received when a child. A kind and concerned teacher in early life may have balanced out a restricting and suppressive father. When we speak from the parent part of ourselves we may find we use such words as 'Why are you so careless?' or 'I am fed up with you always being late' or, if it's from the nurturing parent, 'Come, let me look after you' or 'You poor thing, how difficult it must have been'. A critical parent will adopt a severe facial expression, raise his finger to accentuate his words, usually wear more formal clothes, sit behind a big desk, and adopt a harsh, authoritative voice. A nurturing parent will look at you with concern or provide a shoulder to cry on or a pat on the back. His voice will indicate concern or understanding.

Exercise I

Explore the past week's occurrences and try and remember when you were speaking from the *parent* part of you. Was it the critical or nurturing parent? Do your outward expressions 'mask' the inner parent? Does the 'mask' show an outer parent whereas the 'inner personality' is not feeling at all 'parent-like'?

Adult

The adult part of the personality is the rational, calm and capable part. It solves problems, arrives at decisions, analyses difficulties, determines priorities and does all these tasks in a relaxed and clear manner. We arrive at the adult part of our personality after many life experiences and with various levels of difficulty. Some young children appear to be 'adult' in their behaviour, whilst many adults do not seem to have achieved an inner adult. The inner adult allows us to organise our lives and

145

plan our futures. It is shaped by all sorts of events and continues to develop throughout our lives. Certain mature individuals possess a wisdom which is beyond the reach of most of us and their external behaviour demonstrates a relaxed, peaceful, tranquil pose. They speak slowly and deliberately, check to see if their communication has been understood, appear willing to see both sides of a question, can be assertive but not agressive, can have an air of authority but are not authoritarian, can be calm but are not lazy.

Exercise II

We often choose to 'mask' ourselves with the 'adult' behaviour patterns even though our 'inner personality' may not feel adult. Repeat the exercise in the previous section and list three 'wise' people you are familiar with: with whom you would seek out to discuss a personal problem.

Child

The child part of our personality can be of several kinds. It is the 'needy', 'demanding', 'frustrated' part of ourselves. It can act impulsively, selfishly and occasionally erupt in fury and rage like a baby who has had breast/bottle/toy taken away. On the other hand the child in us may be the appealing, playful, curious, inventive, creative part of our personality. Like a child, it may like to explore and take risks. The child part of our personality reflects how we ourselves were brought up. It can represent both the best and worst of our nature. The 'needy' child will complain – use words like 'I want', 'I must have', 'Why should I', 'It's not fair'. It will appear sullen, with eyes cast down, shoulders drooped. It will sulk, pout, withdraw and occasionally explode in rage. The 'playful' child will laugh, appear relaxed and spontaneous, have a twinkle in its eye, use words like 'terrific', 'wow!' Both the needy and playful child may enjoy touching and hugging and will respond to increased physical contact.

Exercise III

When was the last time you expressed your 'playful' child? How does your 'needy' child express himself and how do you satisfy its needs?

We can now begin to see why so many difficulties arise in communications between two people. If we look at the diagram below, we see that the number of possible combinations is enor-

Figure 1

PERSON A		PERSON B	
INNER PERSONALITY	OUTER PERSONALITY (Mask)	OUTER PERSONALITY (Mask)	INNER PERSONALITY
Critical (P) Nurturing	Nurturing (P) Critical (A) Needy (C) Playful	Nurturing (P) Critical Needy (C) Playful	Critical (P) Nurturing
(A)	Nurturing (P) Critical (A) Needy (C) Playful	Nurturing (P) Critical (A) Needy (C) Playful	(A)
Needy (C) Playful	Nurturing (P) Critical (A) Needy (C) Playful	Nurturing (P) Critical (A) Nurturing (C) Critical	(C)

mous. Not only do we have to be aware of which 'inner person-ality' is communicating but whether we are masking that person-ality with another. For example, I feel very nervous about asking for a rise (inner personality is the needy child). I try and hide this by using the 'critical parent' personality. 'I want a rise or else!' My boss responds with his 'critical parent' personality – 'If you are going to take that attitude . . .' and there goes my rise.

Using the grid to unravel communication difficulties can be very helpful and in transactional analysis this process is taught by the therapist to the clients, e.g.:

In Figure I

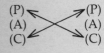

Person (1) says to Person (2), 'What time will you be home tonight?' (It is said from his inner adult with an outer adult expression and vocal tone.) Person (2) replies 'I will be a little late tonight – about 7.30 pm.' (Replies from adult part with adult outer.)

In Figure II

(P) ⟵ ⟶ (P)
(A) ⤬ (A)
(C) ⟵ ⟶ (C)

The same exchange, 'What time will you be home tonight?' is said from the parent part with a critical, blaming expression, directed to person (2) child. Person (2) responds with 'I will be a little late tonight – about 7.30 pm', with irritation and emphasis on the '*little*'. He is replying from his critical parent to the person (1) child.

Eric Berne goes on to explain how when the lines are crossed as in Figure II, misunderstandings, quarrels and miscommunications occur.

It takes a little practice to become familiar with this model. Getting to know your own inner personalities and the 'masks' you choose may help you understand why your relationships develop difficulties. You may be able to identify ways in which your communications can be improved. We will describe some more exercises at the end of this chapter.

One of the consequences that occurs if our inner and outer personalities become limited is that we become fixed in a particular position and adopt an unchanging view of ourselves and of our fellow human beings. These fixed 'life positions' were described by Thomas Harris in his book *I'm OK – you're OK* and they offer a helpful outline for increasing our awareness. These life positions or 'frozen personalities and frozen marks' are:

    (1) I'm OK – You're OK
    (2) I'm OK – Your're not OK
    (3) I'm not OK – You're OK
    (4) I'm not OK – Your're not OK

Position 1 I'm OK – your're OK
In this position, the person feels good about himself. He values his strengths and is aware of his limitatons. He accepts the

necessity to compromise and is able to tolerate uncertainty. He is able to enjoy friendships but is equally content to be on his own. He is content with his lot, at peace with himself and quietly confident. He views the external world and other people with a mixture of interest and tolerance. He accepts other people's failings and is able to separate their actions he dislikes from them as people. He operates mostly from his *adult* but is equally at ease with his *parent* and *child*. He values the *child* part in other people and is not suspicious of their motives.

Position 2 I'm OK – you're not OK

This person operates more from his *parent*. He tends to be critical and judgmental. He can appear smug and superior, arrogant and conceited. His actions may come over in an authoritarian manner and he does not suffer fools gladly. He feels good about himself and may in time learn to feel good about other people. In positions of power and authority he is concerned with plots, coups and sabotage. His *critical parent* may well hide a *needy child*, but once he has accepted the other person he may well shift to position (1).

Position 3. I'm not OK – you're OK

This person sees himself as a victim and is unhappy with his lot. He feels inferior, attempts to buy praise with fawning behaviour and is generally servile and dependent. He mostly operates from his *needy child* and sees other people as possessing a powerful *parent* or *adult*. He is constantly asking for approval and is unable to feel good about himself however much praise he receives. He is happy to allow other people to take advantage of him and will not stand up for himself as he fears rejection. He will seek people in position (2) to reinforce his own fixed position but may shift to position (1) if he feels safe and secure. More often than not, he flips to position (2) when he finds someone who is more 'Not OK' than he is.

Position 4. I'm not OK – you're not OK

This can be the most fixed position. The person feels bad about himself and sees his situation as hopeless and himself as helpless. Not only does he feel a victim but he sees no external source of help. His negativity can take on a forceful expression and he may turn to crime or commit violent acts without any moral qualms. On the other hand he can become very withdrawn and punish himself for the 'sins of the world' that he feels he has caused. In its most extreme form this position requires professional help, which needs to come from someone with extreme patience and sensitivity. One sees this position in children who have been told off – 'Go away, I hate you' – and it is very sad if this stance is retained in adult life.

Examine each of these four positions and see which one describes your most usual stance. We all probably vary from one position to another, but if you find yourself in a fixed position most of the time, then it may be necessary to make a conscious effort to explore how it feels to adopt one of the other positions. Use the following grid to explore how you see your position in the various relationships outlined.

Position	Children	Parents	Friends	Partner	Work Colleagues	Boss
(1) I'm OK – you're OK						
(2) I'm OK – you're not OK						
(3) I'm not OK – you're OK						
(4) I'm not OK – you're not OK						

Families and groups

So far we have described the interactions between two people. When it comes to studying the same process in families or groups the descriptions are more complex and the knots that we manage to tie infinitely more difficult to unravel. One of the major 'balancing acts' we have to perform in our lives is the one between our own individual needs and the needs of the family, group, society or nation we live in. No man is an island, yet living on an island and getting away from it all is a frequent fantasy for all of us. The family unit serves in some way as the transition between the individual's needs and the needs of the group. In all the 4000 societies present on the earth, the family unit forms the base to that society. Experiments with other 'units' such as the kibbutz in Israel or the communes in the United States have generally not developed past their experimental stage. Most of us will have been born into a family (family of origin) and the majority of us will go on to find a mate and create our own family unit. There has been a dramatic decrease in the extended family (more than two generations living together) and even the nuclear family (two parents plus children) has a less frequent pattern than two decades ago. With the increase in divorce, many more single-parent families exist and there has also been an increase in experimental family units with gay men and lesbian women living together and raising their own children.

Each culture has its own pattern of family 'style' but it is possible to detect certain recurring patterns which may help you to identify your own family.

Closed family

In this sort of family the 'rules' are well-known and relatively rigid. 'You brush your teeth every morning before breakfast' or 'No one is to stay out later than 10 pm'. Each family has its own sets of rules, but in a closed family these do not evolve and usually one or other parent is relatively authoritarian. The family appears close-knit and does not accept strangers easily. Attempts by individuals in the family to break out and rebel are usually punished and the family may well collectively side against the rebel and expel him from the family. The rebel may feel rejected, unwanted, and if his attempts to join another unit at school or group at work are similarly unsuccessful he may develop the 'outsider' mentality that has been so well captured by books like *The Rebel* and *The Outsider* (Colin Wilson).

Random family

Here the reverse is true: the family does not have a feeling of being a family, either because of constant conflict between husband and wife or because of a false understanding of the need for permissiveness. Everyone is allowed to do 'their own thing'. The family operates more like a collection of individuals than a unit pulling together. Birthdays and holidays are not jointly celebrated and the rituals and ceremonies present in a closed family are absent. Paradoxically, watching television can help to fragment a closed family but can also bring a random family closer together. Often, watching television together is the nearest a random family gets to having a group ritual.

151

Open family

This is a mixture of these two extremes: the need for individual growth and separateness is recognised whilst at the same time the boundaries of the family group are protected and preserved. Parents learn from their children and alter the family rituals to take into account new interests and new friends, whilst children respect the need to maintain the stability of the family and enjoy continuing the traditions when they form their own families.

The balance between the needs of the individual and the needs of the group (family-community) is mirrored in political attitudes, with one political party stressing the importance of individual freedom and responsibility whilst the other places a great emphasis on central government control and community care. The manner in which we each 'survive' our family of origin and create our own may well influence the pattern of our approach to the political solutions we support.

Family cycle

Like an individual, each family goes through various stages of development, each with its own pleasures and problems. Understanding the ebb and flow of family life may well help prevent the frustration and pain when your own family is under stress or in a crisis. The family of origin is the family you were born into. The first step in creating your own family involves some separation and disengagement either when you leave school or get married. This disengagement process can be made problematic depending on the closeness or randomness of your family of origin. Establishing your own relationship with a fellow human being is the first step in creating your own family unit. How many of your own 'rules' do you bring with you? How does your mate adapt to your style?

In the sections on couples, we looked at the difficulties that occur in relationships and this phase of the family life cycle is where the majority of these issues will first be encountered. This stage may be made more difficult by financial or housing difficulties and if the young couple are still living with either set of parents, being on their own can be made that much more problematic. The next stage involves the arrival of children and for many couples today, with adequate contraception, this stage does not need to coincide with the previous stage. Nevertheless, the arrival of children shifts the focus of the family life from the needs of the adults to those of the young arrivals. Patterns of work, sleep, sex and feeding are usually altered and the young couple begin to develop their own rules and rituals and lay down the foundations for a more or less closed/open-random family.

The next stage involves the children going to school or the wife returning to work or both. Children begin to develop their own personalities, likes and dislikes and the 'family' begins to shape its own characteristics, with decisions on where to go on holiday, how to spend Christmas, who does the washing up, etc. One in four marriages will by now have ended in divorce and the conflicts, pain and distress that result from the break will force both parents and children to face the dissolution of the family unit. How this is handled will be more important than that it has happened. Can the parents avoid blaming each other, especially in front of the children? Can the parents agree to a mutually acceptable 'division'? Will each parent agree to the other visiting and having access? How will they explain the divorce to the children? If there is another person, how much will he or she be involved in caring for the children? The answers to these and many other questions will influence both the children of the first marriage and any children of subsequent marriages. Two in five children now have step-parents, and the complexities of creating a stable family unit in second marriages are even more difficult than in a first marriage.

Having survived this stage and gone back to start again, couples are faced with the children leaving home and the 'empty nest' syndrome. The role the mother has had during the early phases will greatly influence what kind of challenges may have to be faced. This is the time when the man leaves with his secretary or younger woman, leaving a 40–50 year old who has given her life to the family alone, desperate without a job and little identity. It can also be the time when the couple rediscover the joys of being on their own without the demands of children, their home paid for and cared for. They find that being in the company of another human being who has shared a lifetime of pleasure and pain, sorrow and joy, is indeed one of the greatest achievements known to the human species. They approach the next stages of their life together – retirement and the threat of bereavement – with an equanimity found only in those who are at peace, not only with themselves, but with their fellow human beings.

Losing a spouse at this age can be a tremendous blow to either husband or wife and it could be said that the whole of our life so far has been a preparation for this moment. The moment has arrived when we have to let go of a loved one or let go ourselves of our own life. The manner in which we do this is a reflection on the way we have conducted ourselves so far.

Improving your communication

We have already mentioned some of the more general difficulties that arise between people and now will outline a few practical hints on communication.

(1) Increase your own awareness of what it is you want to communicate

This is common sense, but all too often we ourselves are not quite sure what we feel, think, sense (see, hear, touch, smell) and our statements are misunderstood. Be clear whether you want to say something concerning how you

> *Think* – I think you are making the wrong decision
> *Feel* – I felt hurt when you said that
> *Sense* – I saw a bright blue car pass the window

or how you are going to behave.

> *Intention* – I am going to drive the car into the garage.

All too often a 'thinking' statement covers up a 'feeling' state-ment: e.g. 'I think you are making the wrong decision' (I feel very upset you decided to do that); and an 'intention' statement, 'I am going to drive the car into the garage', hides a thinking statement, 'It was stupid of you to leave it out'.

The ability we have to be clear, direct and honest in our own communication will affect how that communication is perceived and responded to. Clarity requires us to be aware of our own 'inner personality', and directness and honesty is a function of how much we are willing or able to reveal about this 'inner personality'. We may be fairly aware but decide to hide behind a mask, or on the other hand be fairly direct and honest but not very aware.

(2) Increase your awareness of what the other person is wanting to communicate

How able are you to listen? Not just with your ears but with your eyes and intuition as well. Allowing the other person to have his say, checking out to see if you have understood ('Now let me get this straight, what you are saying is . . .'), and showing that you have recognised what the other person may be feeling but not wanting to reveal ('It sounds like you were pretty upset when . . .') are all ways of *actively listening* and not just being there with your ears not even opened. We not only communicate with our words but with the gestures, facial expressions, postures and vocal tones we use. If you repeat the sentence 'I want an apple' four times, each time stressing a different word, the message it carries will be different. Improving your communication involves becoming more aware of these non-verbal cues not only from other people but in yourself. Couples who have lived together a long time and have learned how to 'read' the other person extremely accurately, often sit in silence together 'communicating'.

You may need help to improve your communication as it is sometimes difficult to correct a lifetime pattern, let alone be aware of it.

(3) Look after a relationship – do not take it for granted

We all like to be liked, but equally important, we all like to be noticed.

- Let your partner know you appreciate her/him.
- Give positive 'feedback' to someone who has given you pleasure.
- Separate quality time from quantity time (five minutes full attention to a child can be far more important than half-an-hour of ums and ahs).
- Let people know if you have really been upset by something.
- Give yourself enough time if you want to discuss something important.

10

WORKING AND PLAYING

Happiness is not a state one arrives at but the means of travelling. For many people work is seen as the way of earning money, enabling them to live in the style they would like. It is one of the paradoxes of our current economic situation that as many people suffer from the distress of unemployment as suffer from the stress of their work. Somewhere along the line the division between 'work' and 'play' has been so clearly demarcated in our minds that one activity over-determines the other. We cannot 'play' unless we work, but work can be so stressful we are no longer able to enjoy play. And if we have no work, 'play' ceases to have meaning and we find it hard to indulge in it.

The threat of redundancy, the inability to find work, is a devastating experience for many which will affect spirit, mind and body. We derive a sense of identity from our work which is a very necessary part of our self-respect. Unemployment still carries a stigma which suggests laziness and inadequacy, and places the sole responsibility for this state of affairs on the individual concerned. No doubt on occasion this may be so, but for the majority of those out of work, the causes are more complex and are rooted deep in our economic and political systems. The need to provide for oneself and one's family at the most basic level of food, shelter and warmth will almost always override any desire for pleasure, enjoyment and leisure. Nevertheless, whenever one is faced with a life crisis, be it unemployment, a bereavement or a divorce, it is possible to use the opportunity of the changing circumstances to re-examine one's values, direction and purpose. This is not to belittle the necessities of the basic human needs for money, food and shelter, nor to diminish the importance of the emotional turmoil that such a crisis might bring about.

157

Holism implies looking for different levels of meaning arising from one set of 'facts'. No one meaning will completely explain the situation, but each 'level of meaning' will give us a greater understanding of the whole. The way we view our reality may well determine how we respond to it. The 'meaning' can be seen as a pair of spectacles we put on to view the outside world. If we put on a pair of blue spectacles, all we see will be tinged with the colour blue. If we put on a yellow pair, all we see will be yellow, etc. A particularly good example came out of the Vietnam War when doctors discovered that soldiers who had suffered most horrific injuries on the battlefield seemed to be in much less pain than would have been anticipated by the extent of their injuries. It became apparent that for many soldiers, being injured carried with it the likelihood of returning to America. In other words, the 'meaning' they gave to their injuries shaped in some way their responses to them, including the ability to withstand intense pain. So that before we examine in detail some aspects of how work and play impinge on your life, it may be helpful to identify, or bring into greater awareness, your own goals and ambitions for yourself. To do this, it is necessary to explore not only your needs but those of your immediate family and friends. What sort of changes do you anticipate occurring in your life in the next one year, five years, ten years? Let us start by looking at what changes have actually occurred in the past year.

Life Change Index

This Index was developed in 1973 by Holmes and Rahe as a way of measuring the likelihood of health change in individuals. They found that by identifying the number of changes that had occurred in the previous year, they were able to predict the chance of a major health change for that individual. They were also able to identify the degree of stress caused by the stressors and gave each a numerical score. These scores are independent of education, intelligence, sex, race and class. Variations occur between individuals depending on their personal strengths and weaknesses but not between social groups.

LIFE CHANGE INDEX

If an event has been true for you in the past year or will occur in the near future, please mark the space.

Event

Death of spouse	—	100
Divorce	—	73
Marital separation	—	65
Jail term	—	63
Death of close family member	—	63
Personal injury or illness	—	53
Marriage	—	50
Fired at work	—	47
Marital reconciliation	—	45
Retirement	—	45
Change in health of family member	—	44
Pregnancy	—	40
Sex difficulties	—	39
Gain of new family member	—	39
Business readjustment	—	39
Change in financial state	—	38
Death of close friend	—	37
Change to different line of work	—	36
Change in number of arguments with spouse	—	35
Mortgage over £20,000	—	31
Foreclosure of mortgage or loan	—	30
Change in responsibilities at work	—	29
Son or daughter leaving home	—	29
Trouble with in-laws	—	29
Outstanding personal achievement	—	28
Spouse begins or stops work	—	26
Begin or end school	—	26
Change in living conditions	—	25
Revision of personal habits	—	24
Trouble with boss	—	23
Change in work hours or conditions	—	20
Change in residence	—	20
Change in schools	—	20
Change in recreation	—	19
Change in church activities	—	19
Change in social activities	—	18

Mortgage or loan less than £20,000 .... — 17
Change in sleeping habits .... — 16
Change in number of family get-togethers .... — 15
Change in eating habits .... — 15
Vacation .... — 13
Christmas (if approaching) .... — 12
Minor violations of the law .... — 11

                                                                —
                                          Total
                                                                —

Score 150 – gives 50% chance of health change
Score 300 – gives 90% chance of health change

Having identified the actual changes that have occurred, see how well you can anticipate what might occur. For this particular exercise, try to separate what you would like to occur from what you think might actually happen. Use the following outline (table) as a guide for yourself, but you may well find that certain categories important to you are not present.

Question What changes are likely to occur in the following areas in:
  (i) the next one year;
  (ii) the next five years?

ME	FAMILY	FRIENDS	PLAY	WORK	NEIGHBOUR-HOOD
Physical health	Births		Holidays	Promotion	Neighbours
Illness	Deaths		Hobbies	Demotion	Housing
Accidents	Separations	New friends	Interests	Redundancy	Car parking
Operations	Divorces	Old friends	Music	Change of	Library
Exercise	Marriages	Quarrel with	Sport	work	Shopping
Diet	House	friends	Gardening	Change in	Transport
Improve-	change		Reading	salary	Rates
ment in	Mortgage		Television	Change in	Nursery
health	change		Other	work	Local
Menopause	Quarrels			environ-	government
	Sexual			ment	amenities
Mental health	activity			Quantity of	Milkman
Sadness				work	Parks
Happiness				Retirement	Swimming pool

160

ME	FAMILY	FRIENDS	PLAY	WORK	NEIGHBOUR-HOOD
Depression					
Anxiety					
Intimacy					
Aloneness					
Spiritual health					
Sense of purpose					
Sense of direction					
Values					
Beliefs					

Anticipatory planning

Question   What changes are likely to occur in the following areas (for exploration, suggestions):
    (i) in the next one year;
    (ii) in the next five years?

As we have mentioned many times, the purpose of these questionnaires is to increase your own awareness, not necessarily to provide solutions: it is not always possible to provide answers to many of the difficulties facing us, and learning to tolerate uncertainty can be one of the most difficult lessons we have to learn. Carl Jung put it much better when he said:

> The serious problems in life however are never fully solved. If ever they should appear to be so it is a sure sign that something has been lost. The meaning and purpose of a problem seems to be not in its solution but in our working at it incessantly.

There are some problems, however, that we can find solutions to and we can now explore some of these as they relate to work.

Work environment

Occupational health studies have drawn attention to the importance of a number of physical factors which impinge on the place of work. These are *noise – light – temperature – humidity* and *vibration*. The constant ringing of a telephone or a machine, the glare of artificial light and the absence of good ventilation will

161

all increase the level of stress for workers. The recent addition of computers and video display units into offices has introduced a new problem for office workers. Do you have a say in your work environment? Can you alter the place where you sit? Is it possible for you to bring plants or flowers to personalise your own space? Having some degree of control is important for all of us, even if it is only over a small aspect of our work. Look around your place of work and see what changes you can introduce yourself. Even if you work in an automated mechanised factory, it is still possible to retain some individuality. It is the ability to remember your own uniqueness as well as share in the office or factory life that will make your work place less stressful. Find out for yourself what balance feels right.

One aspect of the work environment that is equally if not more important is the other people you work with, especially if you are sharing an office or workroom. Is it possible for you to find some time to be on your own or are you always surrounded? Many work places now operate a 'flexitime' which can give you a few hours to yourself. Whatever the workplace, make sure you give some time to yourself, no matter how demanding the work. If you are answering the telephone, give yourself a few seconds before you pick it up so that it is *you* that decides to answer the phone and not the phone that is dictating to you. When talking on the phone, become aware of the tension in your face and hands, notice what is happening to your breathing and learn to relax whilst working and not just when you get home.

The work itself

Are you in the right sort of job? How much freedom do you have to choose? Does the job have the career prospects that are right for you? Hans Selye, the doyen of stress studies, used to say, 'Find out whether you are a racehorse or you prefer grazing'. If you are ambitious, then a job with no career prospects is not right for you. If you are not ambitious, and there is no reason why you should be, then working in a demanding and pressurised job with good career prospects and a 'rat race' approach to its staff is inappropriate.

Stress at work can come from two areas. There is too much work and the demands made on you are too great. Or the work is beyond your capacity and skills and you may have been promoted to your level of incompetence. The latter dilemma is one that occurs in many businesses, banks and corporations. Because there is a mentality which encourages drive, ambition, performance, it is inevitable that some people will eventually be promoted to a job they are not capable of doing. Saying 'no' to a promotion is difficult but can be essential in saving you from a great deal of unnecessary stress. The corollary to the 'Peter Principle' is that you may be working well below your level of competence. This is particularly true for many women in secretarial or administrative positions who work for incompetent and inefficient executives. Nurses find themselves frustrated by the inadequacies and limited perceptions that many doctors have concerning the 'total' needs of a patient. Because of the hierarchy in the medical profession, nurses find they are unable to influence the care of the patient because the authority for clinical decisions rests with the doctor. Remember, awareness implies being aware of your limitations as well as your strengths.

Whether you are ambitious or not, part of what gives job satisfaction is receiving *feedback*. How well are you doing? Does your employer notice when you work that little bit more or indeed, does he notice when you are away or arrive late? Few employers actually sit down with their employees at the end of the year and tell them how they have done. Getting an honest appraisal of our strengths and weaknesses from someone we trust can be of particular importance and can increase our sense of self-worth. Even if the comments are negative, we have been noticed. People in repetitive factory-line production work can lose their sense of identity and uniqueness because they have in some degree been turned into an extension of the machine they are operating. Seek out 'feedback' whenever you can. Ask for an appraisal of your work: your employer may welcome the opportunity to tell you.

Working with people

Those jobs in which the task involves being responsible for other people carry a particular set of problems and difficulties. Often the individual may have to choose between the job that needs to get done or the individual worker who is going through some personal crisis. Workers in the 'caring' professions – medicine, social work, nursing, counselling etc. – all have to deal with the needs and demands of other human beings who are often in great distress. Doctors and nurses dealing with patients who have a physical infection have learnt the importance of protecting themselves from catching their patient's infections and take precautionary measures (protective clothing, barrier nursing). It is equally necessary for workers involved in dealing with 'psychological distress' to be aware of how infectious that can be. How much 'protection' is it possible to develop without losing the sensitivity, openness and empathy that are necessary tools to continue to work with people?

For many workers in the caring professions this is a constant battle, and an increasing number find themselves requiring counselling, psychotherapy and relaxation to enable them to continue working. The 'burnt-out' syndrome is now a well-recognised fact for many such workers. Doctors have a three times higher rate of alcoholism, suicide and depression than comparable professions and more often than not it is a result of their inability and unwillingness to seek help. The aura of the invincible professional administering to the weak and dependent patient is harmful for both the professional and the worker. The reason why people choose careers in the caring professions may explain why this state of affairs is allowed to continue. There is often an unhealthy collusion between workers and client and an even more unhealthy need on the part of the worker. He may consider that he has been drawn to this profession through a noble and altruistic wish to help the needy. However, on closer examination he may find that he needs the helpless more than the helpless need him. He is then locked into a vicious chain of events that will eventually cause him to face his own need and helplessness. This may manifest itself in many different ways and include the 'burnt-out syndrome'.

The 'burnt-out syndrome' can be prevented by recognising the 'infection' of psychological distress, learning to become aware of the warning signs and taking precautionary measures. Much as the doctor or nurse will wash their hands after examining a patient with an infectious disease, it is important for workers in the caring professions to have some discipline or exercise by which they can psychologically 'cleanse' themselves. Many of the exercises described in this book are ways in which that cleansing can be encouraged.

Another important aspect involved in this sort of work is the ability to say 'No' and mean it. This applies to all aspects of our lives but is of particular importance in the workplace, especially in the caring professions. 'How can I say no to the next demand when I am supposed to care?' 'How can I shut up shop at 5.30

pm when the room is still filled with clients?' 'How can I refuse to attend to a patient even though I have promised to be with the family tonight?' These are all daily dilemmas facing many workers in these professions. Of course it is not always possible so to regulate one's work to pre-empt the emergencies. Nevertheless, planning the week so that one's own needs and wishes receive some recognition is an important way of balancing out the pressures. Cancelling or postponing non-urgent or routine work is not inappropriate following a particularly demanding work routine. Learning to say no to requests for help that can be met by someone else is not unkind or insensitive when you are overworked and stretched to your limit. Encouraging the client/patient to seek solutions for themselves rather than adopting a paternalistic 'there, there, I will take care of it for you', can be protective of your own health and be of more value for the client/patient in the long run.

If you are in a job and are responsible for people but not in a counselling capacity, you may find it difficult to share your own concerns and feelings of insecurity or uncertainty. People in leadership roles often comment on the loneliness and isolation they feel. One of the tasks involved in such a job is making decisions which will not always be approved of by the personnel working for you. Leaders may find the fact that they are not 'liked' difficult to bear. It is part of the function of leadership to accept the 'projections' of the workforce or population. How often does an admired and idealised leader turn into a denigrated and disliked tyrant. If we, as the followers or employees, insist on 'projecting' first of all the positive qualities (leadership, drive, clarity) into our leaders and deny that we have these attributes within ourselves, we shall also end up by 'projecting' the negative qualities (authoritarianism, indecision, uncertainty) into them. Part of the task of a leader is to help his 'followers' to accept responsibility for these projections, whilst at the same time accepting that he may indeed have greater drive, clarity etc.

Women and work

One of the major social changes that has occurred in the last thirty years has been the alteration in patterns of work for women. Women have always worked, but only recently have they been more fairly paid for it. Up until the beginning of this century the work involved household activities and menial

165

factory work. The woman professional worker is a very recent development in our society and the notion that women have a right to careers, promotion and professional development is still a fairly new concept. However, there is an increasing number of careers now open to women even though men still appear to inhabit the top posts in most professions.

For women the problems start from birth with the biased educational system and the lack of adequate role-models. Having struggled to university, many women will find a major hurdle in competing with their male colleagues for jobs. In spite of the Equal Opportunities Act, many employers will select men in preference to women and promotion will also be harder. On average, men earn £10 to every £6 earned by women and it is not difficult to see why women are the largest group discriminated against in our society. Even in the professions of law, medicine, teaching and social work, the majority of top posts are held by men and there are still too few women in political psitions.

The major reason given for this is that the traditional division of labour – the man going out to work and the woman staying and looking after the home – has served us well for centuries and helps to stabilise our society and protect family life. This may well have been so in previous generations, but only 10% of current family units are the traditional father-mother-two children. The majority of the population live in different units, including single parents, childless marriages, second and third marriages, widowed and extended family units. In these units, the need for the woman to be in paid employment is often necessary, not only for economic reasons. Modern electrical appliances have made the job of looking after a home that much easier and the need for all of us to have a sense of identity is reinforced by having a job or profession.

Nevertheless, many women still will have to face the difficulty of deciding between career and home. Putting off the decision until the late 20s or early 30s can make the problem eventually more difficult. The solution for many need not be as starkly portrayed – it does not have to be either career or home, and there are several options that it is helpful to have considered. Needless to say, the discussions and decisions should be arrived at jointly and with as much awareness of what the consequences might be.

Each of these decisions will have its advantages and disadvantages and not one is the perfect solution. What is important is that it is arrived at with proper discussion and awareness of all the issues including the financial consequences. Some women will feel guilty because they are working and having the children at home, others will feel guilty because they are not using their degree or do not contribute financially to the household. Guilt is almost inevitable but mostly unnecessary and certainly unhelpful.

Career/Home – possible options
- decide on career and have no children
- decide to stay at home in early years and resume later on
- employ child-minder/nursery/au pair/nanny
- job-share with mate
- job-reversal with mate
- work from home
- part-time work
- decide you enjoy being a live-in wife and mother and stay at home

---

Having decided to work, women will then face difficulties not usually encountered by men. The issue of equal pay and promotion has already been mentioned, but even more distressing is sexual harassment. Surveys suggest that this is far more common than is acknowledged and will range from a suggestive comment or look to an actual assault. Looking sexy at work is often encouraged in certain offices and professions, and women can unwittingly be led into being treated as sex objects. Natural timidity and fear of losing one's job often prevent women from protecting themselves and taking the necessary precautionary steps.

Some women, encouraged by the feminist movement, have taken an assertive and aggressive response to unwanted sexual advances. This may provoke an even more aggressive reply on the part of the male, but it is a strategy well worth considering, especially if other people are present. This particular strategy (assertive or aggressive response) is one which some women are concerned may creep into their general stance towards life if they pursue their ambitions. Indeed, one of the consequences of the feminist movement has been the 'masculisation' of women who have learnt to adopt the strategies usually employed by men. In men, they can be seen as driving, forceful, determined

– in women, the same responses could be seen as strident, aggressive and castrating. Women who want to get to the top and do not want to lose their 'feminity' have to struggle with men and women who will judge their normal ambitions and drives in a prejudicial manner.

11

YOU AND YOUR ENVIRON-MENT

The holistic approach concerns itself with how 'parts' affect the whole and how the 'whole' affects the parts. So far, we have been talking about parts of us – body-mind-spirit – but each one of us is part of a larger whole – our families – and each family is part of a small community, and each community is part of a nation, and so on. As human beings, we form only a small, but nevertheless very important part of all the animal life present on the earth. We have been labelled the most dangerous species in the world because our potential for destructiveness has been so obvious. To list the way we have over the centuries polluted our rivers, destroyed our wildlife and rendered many other species extinct would be a depressing and painful activity. Depressing because it would highlight the total lack of concern and awareness we exhibit as to the effect we have on our environment, and painful because it would underline our collective stupidity. As we sow, so shall we reap, and many of the concerns, distresses, diseases and epidemics affecting us at this stage of our progress are the direct result of the influence of the environment on us.

Fortunately, in the last twenty or thirty years there has been an increased focus on the way the environment affects the health of the individual. Just as we need to increase our awareness of the interconnectedness between body, mind and spirit, so we need to understand how each of our actions, from smoking a cigarette to throwing a can of beer away, affects our fellow human beings, some of them many thousands of miles away, others our neighbours in our street. Ecology, conservation, preservation, Friends of the Earth, Greenpeace, are all words and causes more in the news than twenty years ago. For some, they carry the message of 'doom and gloom', and are dismissed as unhelpful and cranky. For others, they are seen as the watchdogs of the future, a future which for many may not exist if we do not begin to address ourselves to the relationship between the individual and the environment. In the context of this book, we shall focus on some of the very practical aspects of daily living as they affect health, but in the process it is necessary to remember the reasons why this is important.

One of the basic Hippocratic principles of good health was that health could only be achieved by living in accordance with natural laws, in such a way that body, mind and spirit maintained a harmonious equilibrium with the total environment.

Awareness has been a constantly recurring theme. A second one would be *balance* – finding the right balance between the needs of the individual (freedom of choice, sense of control) and that of the group (concern for stability and adequate sharing of resources). Finding the right balance in our lives between the need to be alone and the need to be in the company of others, finding the balance between healthy nationalism and appropriate internationalism.

Man's concern with the environment is not new – soil erosion concerned Plato in 400 BC as it also brought down the Mayan civilisation in Central America in 900 AD. Hunting was prohibited in the Royal Parks – a rather self-interested conservation law. Many so-called 'primitive' tribes in North America and the Far East lived according to the laws of Nature, and were, and still are, appalled by the 'white man's' disregard for the fundamental principles of preservation and conservation. The industrial society brought many benefits to mankind but in its trail it has left us with a legacy of industrial diseases. The smog in London in 1952 was responsible for over 4,000 deaths and the Clean Air Bill passed in 1954 was a first step in the politicisation of environmental causes.

During the 1960s, a series of books began to have an impact on people's awareness and the 'modern' environmental-ecological movements date from those times. These books included *Silent Spring, Only One Earth, Population Bomb, Limits to Growth, Spaceship Earth*. They all drew attention to different aspects of the effect we were having on the environment from the use of pesticides and air pollution to the effects of overpopulation and the danger of the nuclear holocaust. Many of the wilder predictions in these seminal books have since proved to be wrong, but they served as 'warning signs' for us all. The Brandt Commission in 1980 brought together many of these concerns and placed them within the context of the relationship between the developed nations (north) and the underdeveloped (south). The problems as seen by the various studies can be summarised by saying that we in the north overconsume (food, energy, raw materials) and waste (food, energy, raw material). This overconsumption and wastage in the industrialised north (one-fifth of the world's population) adds to the overpopulation and malnutrition of the south.

It is quite understandable that when presented with such global descriptions of the problems, individuals will say, 'Well, what can I do?' Personal sacrifices seem pointless in the midst of such vast waste. The most anyone can do, and that is not to belittle the gestures, is to donate to charities and hope that someone else will deal with the problem. The two hurdles that have to be overcome are, first, the lack of awareness and secondly, the feeling that one's individual efforts are not important. This issue is not a question of how your individual effort affects the starving millions, but of how your individual effort affects you. Looking after your own environment will help make you aware of the interconnectedness and encourage the balance and harmony necessary for your individual health. For the purposes of this chapter, we have excluded other people as part of your environment as we have dealt with this area in the chapter on relationships.

You make connections with your environment through your five senses (sight, hearing, touch, taste and smell). In addition, your five orifices (mouth, nose, penis/uretha/vagina, anus, skin pores) allow you to eat, speak, spit, vomit, breathe, urinate, ejaculate, give birth, defecate and sweat. It is an unusual way to look at aspects of pollution and conservation, but it does allow for individualising these issues and reducing them to the question, 'What can I do about my immediate environment?'

The following questions may provide you with some answers to this:

Sight
Look around your home – what do you use, how would you describe the inside of your cupboards or your fridge? What would a total stranger be able to say about you from looking at your garden? Do you have house plants? The actual content of the inside of your house will obviously vary from culture to culture, economy to economy, and each of us will have our own

preferred 'style'. Many will be limited by financial constraints, but how have you arrived at a balance between tidiness and untidiness? Is your house full of 'consumer' items? Is there a focal point to the house? Is there a quiet place? What things can you do to make it look in keeping with your current needs?

Next time you go out, take a look at your road and immediate neighbourhood. What eyesores are there? What would the insides of your dustbins tell someone about the problems of consumption and waste in your own household? We use electricity to enhance our sight. How much lighting is really necessary at night? Review the way you light up your home and examine what can be switched off. Television does not consume all that much electricity, but how much of your energy does it consume? Be far more determined over what you choose to watch. Experiment by not having the television on for at least one day a week.

Our eyes will allow us to look at our environment. Looking at the countryside or the seaside is a major leisure pursuit for many of us. Looking at the countryside closely will reveal the ravages we have inflicted on it – the disappearing hedges, the wildlife in danger of extinction, the voluminous evidence of our 'throwaway' society. Conservation of the countryside begins with conservation of your own little bit, be it a window box, a patch-size garden or your local park.

Sound

What noises might be heard coming from your home? How do you speak to your family and friends? Can you tell when your voice is raised? Is there laughter in your life? What music do you like and do you allow yourself to hear it? Is there a time for 'no sound'? Experiment with having a meal a week in silence. What sounds do you hear on being silent? Do you long for someone to speak with? Additions to sound come from radios and television at home, and having noisy neighbours can be one of the most irritating environmental health hazards possible. Do you know if you make too much noise for your neighbour's comfort? Ask them. Is there a squeaky door or a cupboard that rattles in your kitchen? It is often these small, constant stressors in the background that can provide the 'last straw'. A major 'sound stressor' is the telephone. If you are overburdened, take the telephone off the hook for a few hours.

172

Touch

What does your handshake feel like? Ask someone. When was the last time you hugged someone? Do you like being touched? Through the sense of touch, we feel hot and cold. What is the temperature in your household? How much do you know about conservation and heat preservation? Is your loft insulated (30–40% heat loss can be reduced through good insulation and lagging). Double glazing will save a considerable amount on fuel bills. Do you really need to heat every room in the winter?

An extension of touch is what touches us – soap, bathing and showers and clothes. We each use on average 125 litres of water a day. Having a shower instead of a bath not only conserves energy in terms of heating but reduces water consumption (80 litres for a bath, 24 litres for a shower). A shower can be invigorating and raise your own energy level, whereas a bath can help to relax and put you to sleep. If you can, experiment with both.

We cover our bodies with clothes and many, many millions of pounds are spent on the manufacture and purchasing of clothes. Fashion dictates we change our clothes, not when they have worn out, but when we get tired or bored with them, or because we want to maintain our credibility with our friends. Change is necessary and should be looked for, but watch how often you dispose of items from your wardrobe because you want to purchase a new 'set'.

Taste

The chapter on diet explores this area in greater depth, but remind yourself that the major problem in the western world is that we eat too much and waste an even greater amount. Sugar is probably the greatest taste addition for most people and our consumption of sweets, biscuits, cakes, pastries, fizzy drinks, ice lollies, chocolates, together with their attendant packages of cellophane wrappers and aluminium cans (on average we each use the equivalent of 1000 soft drink cans a year), is enough to provide for the needs of many of our less-privileged citizens. Accompanying this increase in our consumption of refined carbohydrates (sugar products) come the diseases of western civilisation – coronary artery disease, diabetes, gall stones etc. Our senses generally determine much of the food industry's patterns of production and manufacture. There is a popular misconception that protein can only be obtained from meat and fish. Not only do we eat more protein than we need, but the source of protein determines the pattern of our agricultural industry. Two-thirds of all the protein eaten in the world is derived from vegetable sources (grains, beans, vegetables). Meat requires 10 units of energy input to provide 1 unit of energy for the consumer, whereas rice provides 40 units of energy for the consumer and requires only 1 unit of energy to do so.

Food	Energy input	Energy output
	By farmer	To consumer
Meat	10	1
Fish	100	1
Wheat	1	3
Rice (intensive farming)	1	40

Insisting that our applies look like 'apples' means that we wax them. Requiring the 'right' colour requires colouring. We eat the equivalent of over 20 tablets of aspirins in food additives a day and more than half of them are for purely cosmetic reasons. The overconsumption leads to forced feeding and the increased use of pesticides and chemical fertilizers. Check all the items of food you buy for the list of additives and see if you can avoid purchasing them. Not only will you aid your own health but you will ensure that food manufacturers get the message. Food is packaged in paper, cans, bottles: all these items are recyclable and your local community may well have a recycling scheme – try and use it.

Smell

We have in some ways tried to eliminate 'natural smells' from our lives and spend a large amount of money on disinfectants, deodorants, perfumes, after-shaves and aerosol sprays. The sensitivity of our sense of smell has become blunted and we no longer consider it to be an important link with our environment. Yet bad smells from decomposing food or blocked drains can be an important environmental hazard. Because we over-consume, we increase our garbage. Each household throws away about 30 lbs of garbage a week. Without too much difficulty, this can be reduced by half and many local communities and big cities have achieved that reduction in a relatively short space of time.

Breath/air pollution

We have constantly underlined the importance of breathing and focussed mostly on how we breathe. Breathing connects us with each and every other human being in the world. Because of airflow, winds and currents, it is possible to calculate that in every breath of air we inhale there will be one million atoms that have been breathed at some time by every other human being on this planet. We do indeed live in a participatory universe and one of the benefits of television and satellite communication has been to increase the sense of the universality of human experience.

The quality of the air we breathe is as important as how we breathe, and that quality is affected by our own personal habits (smoking, driving, burning fuel) as well as our industries. It is now increasingly unacceptable to smoke in public places, lead-free petrol is now the rule in the United States, and since 1958 Londoners have had 70% more sunlight in December because of the Clean Air Act. Nevertheless, in the last ten years we have reaped the consequences of our past profligacy, and acid-rain has killed off half the fish in the lakes of Ontario, destroyed acres of forest, defaced many of our public buildings and corroded miles of railway tracks. This is the direct consequence of our coal burning, sulphur dioxide-producing habits, both personal and industrial. It is not good enough to expect the government to take the necessary steps if we are not prepared to exercise the appropriate control.

Transport

When we want to explore our environment, we need transport and our modern way of life allows us to travel many more miles than our grandfathers ever did. In 1914, the average American male travelled 1640 miles a year, of which 1300 were on foot. In 1970, this figure is 10,000 miles a year, the majority of which is in a car or by an aeroplane. Our transport needs are made possible by the motor car, public transport systems and commercial airlines. In the not too distant future, some of us will become space travellers. 90% of all motor travel is by private car. This produces the familiar traffic jam and air pollution in most of our busy cities. Riding a bicycle to work may decrease your use of a car, may increase the exercise you take, but you will be subject to the fumes of all your fellow car travellers. Yet somehow we do need to rationalise our transport system. The demise of the railway from 4200 to 2400 railway stations in twenty years and the decrease in bus journeys only mean more individual cars with the attendant pressure on our roads. Again, individual decisions by us can affect the quality of life not only for ourselves but for our fellow citizens.

Community

Underlying much of what we have said is the balance we choose to make between looking after ourselves – 'I'm all right Jack' and looking after others. It is apparent, however, that altruism and selfless behaviour on our part has a way of rebounding and rewarding us in ways that may not be immediately obvious. Making the connections with the environment will increase the sense of belonging and will decrease the sense of isolation and loneliness. Getting away from your home and immediate environment will take you into your local community. A well-knit community will be able to withstand many of the pressures both from outside (natural disasters, threat from other communities) as well as from the inside (unemployment, local crime). Tragedies like the Aberfan disaster or the famine in Ethiopia illustrated how the powerful forces within the community surfaced to help cushion the blow for the individual members.

What are the aspects of your own local community that may be important to you? Being aware of your local library, parks and sports amenities may affect you directly. How accessible is your doctor's surgery or local hospital? Your local council will be responsible for schools, nurseries and residential homes for the elderly. How well do you know your local voluntary agencies? Is there a branch of Age Concern, or Oxfam, or the NSPCC in your area? Has your local police station reintroduced community beats, and do you know your local bobby? Those communities that have started a neighbourhood watch scheme have experienced a 30–40% fall in crime rate – has yours? You may not be a churchgoing person, but nevertheless you almost certainly will find one local group that appeals to you. Again, you may not wish to be an active member, but joining and possibly donating either some money or some of your time, or jumble, will be one way of increasing your involvement with your local community.

Many self-help groups now exist to provide support, comfort and information for people with a particular disease or disability – Arthritis Care or Cancer Link. Your local community health councils represent the consumer voice. They can act on your behalf if you have any particular problem or complaints with the Health Service. Make a balance sheet between what you get out of your local community services and what you put in – other than taxes! Expecting 'the council' or the 'government' to provide everything is as unbalanced as expecting everyone to 'stand on their own two feet'. The question is not about supply and demand or dependency and independence but more about interdependence.

We have strayed into the area of politics and it may appear as if this is not an appropriate topic for a book on health. Yet we have seen how many of the factors affecting the choices we make about our food, air, shelter, access to doctors, hospitals, drug costs etc. are all essentially political decisions. How do we arrive at the political 'spectacles' we wear, and how do these political spectacles affect our perceptions? It would be odd indeed if a book on holistic living excluded *the* most important aspect affecting our lives today – the nuclear debate. Not only does the use of nuclear energy affect our environment but the threat of nuclear war is critical to our survival.

Nuclear energy as fuel

Man's need for a reliable energy source accelerated tenfold with the onset of the industrial revolution. Coal, oil and gas (fossil fuels) were all separately developed to provide fuel for electricity generating boards to run our industries, cars and home appliances. With the advent of the atom bomb in 1945, many scientists worked towards putting the 'atom to peaceful work'.

The first nuclear power plant was built at Harwell and since then another twelve have been built together with the attendant research and scientific bases. The original nuclear power stations are now being replaced by the fast breeder reactors, and because the latter are designed to run on *plutonium* and not uranium like the original power stations, they are theoretically self-supporting (they produce more plutonium than they consume). In a nuclear power station, the heat from the fission (atom splitting) is used to boil water to steam which then powers the generator creating electricity.

The advantages of nuclear power are many, but so are the disadvantages. Not least is the fact that it is very difficult to separate the question of nuclear energy as a fuel from the use of nuclear energy for armaments. These industries have developed side by side and are closely interdependent. It was thought that the peaceful use of nuclear power could expand to countries which do not want to have the bomb. Yet some of these countries, such as India, Israel and Iraq, have developed nuclear fuel and it is estimated that several other countries will have a nuclear bomb in the next few years. The non-proliferation treaty does not seem to have succeeded in its intentions.

NUCLEAR POWER

Advantages	Disadvantages
Cheap	Human factor
Unlimited supply	Problem of waste storage
Not labour intensive	Link with arms race
Greater yield than coal or oil	Melt down
Not reliant on foreign countries	Leakage
'Protects' fossil fuel sources	Terrorism
'Independent of union militancy'	
'Safe' (few industrial accidents, unlike coal or oil)	

In addition, in the last few years we have had a series of accidents – Three Mile Island, Windscale, Chernobyl – which have increased the level of concern. The problem with nuclear power stations is that although they may well be 'clean' and 'safe' in comparison with the coal or oil industry, if an accident were to occur the casualties would be horrendous and the effects on the environment long-lasting. It is these horrendous effects of the nuclear explosion that are put to use in the atomic, hydrogen and neutron bombs.

Effects of nuclear explosion
The atom bombs dropped on Hiroshima and Nagasaki killed 130,000 and 70,000 people respectively. The Hiroshima bomb

(Little Boy) was equivalent to 12.5 kilotons of TNT and the one at Nagasaki (Fat Man) to 22 kilotons of TNT. The US and USSR have between them warheads able to deliver the destructive power of 20,000 megatons or 1.5 million Hiroshimas. A nuclear bomb able to be stored under a bed has more destructive power than all the explosives used in the Second World War. The effects of a nuclear explosion have been relatively well documented and studied. The destructive effects result from the intense light, heat and 'blast' as well as the immediate and long-term effects of nuclear radiation. The psychological damage for those who survived the Japanese explosions is still being encountered.

In 1982 the British Medical Association produced a report on the medical effects of nuclear war in Britain and its conclusions were that given the predicted level of attack, none of the precautionary measures – evacuation, shelters and early-warning systems – would prevent the consequences. It felt that these were of such a high level that no possible medical planning would be of any help. It is clear from reading this and other reports that in the event of a nuclear war, survival is not an option we are likely to experience. Of course we may have to face a melt-down in a nuclear reactor, a human accident or a terrorist threat. In each of these instances the destruction would not be total and many of the Civil Defence and Home Office directives would be helpful and necessary. However, it is clear that the only solution to the possibility of a nuclear holocaust is to focus on preventon rather than treatment after it happens.

The possibility of a nuclear war brings along with it the likelihood of destruction of the human species. It is *the* greatest threat to health facing us today. In comparison to this threat, all others pale into insignificance. We do not have to be politically active to appreciate the importance of this threat, but if the basis to the holistic approach is increasing our awareness of ourselves and our environment, it would make no sense if we were to avoid highlighting this issue and discussing the various alternatives that have been put forward by politicians, scientists, environmentalists, as well as philosophers, historians and spiritual leaders. No one in our society today can afford not to have an opinion on this question.

The nuclear debate
It seems that the various proponents in this debate fall into one

of three camps. The first are the proponents of the *deterrent* theory, the second the *disarmers*, and the third group, probably the majority, have no fixed view but are willing to allow the politicians to deal with the dilemma. 'I won't be around to worry, so why should I care?' It is interesting to observe how the first, second and third groups respectively take up a *fight*, *flight* and *flow* response to the threat of nuclear war as a stressor. Unfortunately, none of these responses appears to provide the solution as none helps to recreate a stable balance. Let us look at each in turn.

Deterrent (fight response)

This argument is based on the belief that it is a less evil option and that it has worked for 40 years, i.e. there has not been a nuclear holocaust because the other side knows that it would be destroyed as well if one were to occur. It is therefore important to ensure that the other side appreciates that we are not bluffing and that it is essential to keep our armaments up-to-date and keep matching fire-power with fire-power. The argument goes on to describe why disarming would in fact bring about a greater likelihood of a nuclear holocaust and eventual domination by 'the other side'. Some proponents would go so far as to say that we need to elevate the 'fight response' to a first-strike option. The moral basis to this argument is that we are facing an evil and tyrannical enemy, that we are justified in using all our efforts to destroy it. In other words, we are fighting a 'just war', and morally the evil of using nuclear weapons is less than the evil of not using them.

Disarm (flight response)

The disarmers would start by arguing that the logic supporting the deterrent's case is false and that the end result of the nuclear arms race is an inevitable war. They draw on the testimonies of many retired service officers, scientists and philosophers to support their case. They point out the increasing likelihood of an accident or computer failure and argue that since several other countries now possess the bomb (India, Pakistan, Israel, South Africa), the logic of deterrence no longer holds. Moreover, the possibility of a terrorist outrage with nuclear weapons can no longer be excluded. Their view is that only by disarming, either nationally or globally, will the risk of nuclear warfare be diminished and that someone must give the lead. Some would go so far as to say 'better red than dead', which I suppose is the ultimate flight response, just as 'better dead than red' is the ultimate fight response.

The moral argument for disarming is based on the idealist position that there is never any justification for the use of nuclear weapons – in other words, one can never fight a just war with the bomb. The supporters of the deterrent would adopt a more realist position and argue that it is the lesser of two evils. They would also point out that we cannot turn our back on the nuclear age, and that disarming and destroying our nuclear expertise goes against all we know about our evolution as species.

Devolutioners (flow response)

CND – the Campaign for Nuclear Disarmament – has experienced a revival in Britain and in the last few years we have witnessed many large demonstrations on the part of the disarmers. Nevertheless, the vast majority of the population either prefer not to dwell on this subject or, if they do, find it impossibly difficult to reach any conclusions. The majority will be content for the debate to be carried on by others and devolve their own responsibility when faced with these enormous questions. Every five years, at election time, they will weigh up the pros and cons of the differing viewpoints and make a decision. On that evidence, it appears that the majority support a 'deterrent' approach and feel suspicious and unhappy about the disarmers' case. Whether this decision is arrived at consciously or is a result of accepting the status quo, i.e. flowing with the prevailing approach, it is difficult to determine. What seems to be true is that we may not have the luxury of waiting every five years for decisions of this magnitude to be made. The time-scale and pace of the nuclear arms race is such that we need to ensure that the debate is constantly in our awareness.

Suggested guidelines for a holistic approach to the environment

- Eat less protein (reduce meat, or change your source of protein)
- Walk to the shops
- Take your own carrier bag with you when shopping
- Look out for additives labelled on consumable purchases

- Insulate your home when possible
- Hang a curtain behind your front door in the cold weather
- Switch off one unnecessary light at night
- Repair and mend when you can
- Recycle where possible – cans
  - paper
  - bottles
- Make a compost heap with vegetable waste
- Avoid pesticides, sprays or chemical fertilizers
- Reduce the use of aerosols
- Do not smoke in public places
- Join one local community group
- Join one national community group
- Make yourself familiar with the nuclear debate

12

ABOUT TIME

One of the most frequent statements we hear from patients attending our classes is, 'I have no time' for all this relaxation or jogging or paying more attention to diet. Like the environment around us, time is an aspect of our lives that we seldom pay attention to. Nevertheless it plays an important part in our perception of ourselves and the way we handle the stressors present in our lives. We may occasionally worry about aspects of our environment, like pollution or noise, but we rarely concern ourselves with the relationship we have with time. Yet time can become a major stressor, either because we have too much of it on our hands and are bored or conversely, like the White Rabbit, are constantly referring to our watches and attempting to catch up with ourselves. Time is something we take for granted, a bit like the sky or the sun. It was there before we were born and will be there after we die. However, unlike the sun and the sky, we cannot accurately 'see' time, nor can we hear it or smell it. Yet having an accurate 'sense of time' can be critical not only for telling jokes and in communication generally but for business and professional reasons. We are aware of people who are governed by time and are impatient if they are kept waiting a few minutes. Others seem to have no sense of time and are always late. Yet others are persecuted by time and feel overwhelmed by the demands placed on them and are constantly delaying and dithering, refusing to make a decision, saying, 'It's not the right time'. Most people who are told they have a terminal illness, immediately want to know 'How much time do I have', and we could go on and on.

It is only fairly recently that we have begun to study more carefully the influence of time on health and more specifically the body's physiological processes. We now know for instance that blood pressure, pulse rate, hormone levels, sleep patterns and several other physiological activities have their own 'inner clock' which does not always follow the outer clocks on our wrists or mantlepieces. With the advent of transatlantic flights we have become familiar with 'jet lag' and the feelings of listlessness, disorientation and distress that accompany too rapid a change between our internal and external clocks. For many years menstrual periods have been known to be affected by the moon cycle, and the notion that the 'full moon' affects mental stability has now been relatively well documented. Air hostesses frequently lose their periods as they travel backwards and forwards over the time barrier. Several physicians now feel that some of the illnesses present in our civilisation today are the direct result of the disturbance in the relation to 'time' that has occurred especially in the last fifty years.

Experience of time

Our forefathers, before clocks were invented, saw time as a cyclical phenomen. They observed the sun rising and setting, the moon going through a cycle of new moon to full moon and the seasons changing from spring through to winter and back to spring again. Time was worshipped as a god and was often depicted as a river or ocean encircling the earth. Time was seen to flow but had neither beginning nor middle or end – it was a mixture of all three and what once was the end became the beginning and so on. This notion of *cyclical* time is well described by poets and mystics and one of the characteristics of the mystical or spiritual experience is its 'timelessness' – time stood still. The mystical state has been called the timeless moment.

Blake wrote:

> I see the past present and future
> existing all at once before me.

Eliot, in his amazing work *Four Quartets*:

> Time present and time past
> Are both perhaps present in time future
> And time future contained in time past.

And found scribbled on a lavatory wall was this equally perceptive graffito:

> Time is nature's way of keeping everything
> from happening at once.

With the advent of instruments to measure time following Huygens' invention of the pendulum clock in the seventeenth century, our perception of time began to change. From having a circular relationship with time, we began to have a *linear* one. We began to see the past, present and future all strung out in a line with the past occurring before the present and the future occurring after the present. The idea that this concept of time is 'new' and somehow not real is particularly difficult to grasp intellectually and many reading this will initially dismiss the challenge to this idea of time as ridiculous. Before we go on to try and explain why this is not irrational let us look more closely at our subjective experience of time.

Although there have been numerous attempts to identify a sense-organ in the body that perceives time, as the ear perceives sound, no clear evidence has as yet come to light. Some authorities believe the pineal gland, a small sliver of neural tissue, is the possible location. Our time sense, though, does appear to be measurable and can be altered by specific external factors, e.g. drugs or deprivation chambers. Taking marijuana or LSD alters the perception of time and subjects describe having lost their sense of time, and when asked to estimate the time they have been 'high' are hopelessly inaccurate, either lengthening or shortening the time. Having a temperature can alter your subjective sense of time as measured against an 'objective' clock. But which is 'right' – if you think that time is going slowly, does that occur or is the objective clock time the accurate indicator of 'time'? Is there such a thing as objective time that is out there to be measured and does not change? The discrepancy between our inner subjective clocks and our outer objective clocks produces both physiological (body) and psychological (mind) conflict. This conflict has accelerated since Descartes, for reasons we have explained.

Do we eat when we are hungry and sleep when we are tired or when the external clock time tells us it is the right 'time to eat'? Some people are notorious 'owls', being able to stay up well into the night, whereas others are 'larks', able to get up early in the morning and dropping off to sleep after 9 pm. The balance we maintain between the rhythm of our 'inner clock' and that of our 'outer clock' will affect the relationship we have with time. In other words, our relationship to time affects the way we perceive the external world (observe your response next time you are late for work) and the external world affects the way we perceive time (observe your 'sense of time' on the next occasion you are sitting in the countryside or by the sea). The 'relative' nature of time was finally demonstrated by Einstein in his classic experiments at the beginning of this century. We have still not caught up with the implications that his discoveries have on health and illness. Einstein, in the humourous way found in all great geniuses, described his notion of time in the following way:

> If you sit with a beautiful girl two hours may seem
> like two minutes.
> If you sit on a hot stove two minutes may seem
> like two hours.

Time sickness

How can we translate these last few paragraphs into practical guidelines for daily living? What we are saying is that *if we artificially accelerate our biological clocks we run the risk of developing time sickness*. Time sickness can show itself in many different ways, from 'time-relaxed anxiety' which produces a feeling of being overwhelmed, leading to irritability, inability to relax and competitiveness, to effects on blood pressure, heart-rate, blood cholesterol and hormonal changes. The constellation of these effects is found in those people labelled 'A' type personality. They have a greater incidence of heart attacks and their accelerated inner time clock leads them to an 'untimely' early death. They rush through their 'allotted three score years and ten' in fifty or even forty years. Freidman and Roseman, the cardiologists who first described the 'A' type personality, had their attention drawn to this possibility by an upholsterer. He had been asked to re-cover the seats of the chairs in their waiting room which had become worn. He noticed that the chair seats were only worn on the edge of the seats. The patients waiting to see the cardiologists were so 'busy' and worried about 'time' that they literally sat on the edge of their seats.

Time sickness, or hurry sickness, is a relatively new disease unrecognised as yet by many doctors. The 'treatment' is somehow to alter the inner clock and help it to slow down. The relaxation and meditation exercises described in the previous chapter are increasingly being prescribed for such individuals. These exercises allow us to develop mastery over the 'pace' of our inner clocks. As we slow down both physically and mentally, so we reverse the process that we unwittingly allowed ourselves to get into. Developing some control over our inner clock will allow us also to accelerate it when we need to. If we are suddenly faced with a major demand or fall behind in our allotted tasks, then being able to switch to fourth gear or over-drive may be very necessary. Successful and capable people who get to the top of their professions are those who know how to slow down as well as when to accelerate.

So far we have referred to time and its relation to our daily experience. The intervals we have been focussing on have been hours, days, weeks and months. Let us now turn to some of the longer intervals of time and examine how they can affect our well-being.

The seven seasons

One of the many myths of human development has been that because physical growth stops at about 18–19, psychological growth also ceases. Many of the stories we are fed on as children end with early adulthood – 'they got married and lived happily ever after'. The idea that 'adults' change and continue growing has been one of the fundamental beliefs of the 'growth move-ment' that has been of such great influence in psychotherapy and adult education in the last thirty years. There have been many excesses committed by people in the name of 'individual growth' and we have already mentioned the danger of narciss-istic self-absorption with the accompanying loss of a sense of responsibility to the group or society. Nevertheless, many adults have been freed to explore aspects of their personality and seek answers to questions that have led man to greater awareness and maturity.

The concept of different tasks at different developmental stages is of course not new and Shakespeare was not the first to refer to 'the seasons in a man's life'. Jung constellated his own beliefs into the statement that the first half of life, 0–40, has to do with exploring and coming to terms with our external world of school, jobs, family and citizenship and the second half of life, 40–80, has to do with exploring our internal world. This involves seeking answers to the perennial questions that men have asked – Who am I? What is life all about? What is the purpose of my life? etc. Jung felt that all the problems he encoun-tered amongst his patients over the age of 40 were essentially spiritual ones and he was one of the most important western

187

explorers of our inner world. Referring back to the concept of cyclical time, it is possible to portray our lives as having springs, summers, autumns and winters irrespective of age or stage. Many of us will have known very bleak and cold periods of our lives whereas it is at times possible to recollect phases where everything we touched was successful and grew and blossomed. Sometimes the seasons appear to have got stuck and it may feel as if our lives are a perpetual winter with no spring or summer. It is possible to find both positive and negative attributes to every season. Winter can be welcoming and associated with warm fires and cosy chats, whereas spring can be chaotic and confusing as all the energy seems uncontainable. Which is your favourite season? How would you describe the current phase in your life?

A cyclical view of time suggests that there is a return to the beginning each time, with little or no progress, whereas a linear view suggests an ever upward and onward development, with stagnation or reversal appearing as failure. If we combine the two symbols of a circle and a line, we get a spiral. This symbol may be a more accurate description of our relationship to time.

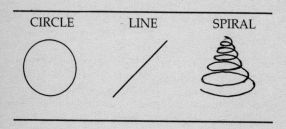

Like a mountain traveller we circle the mountain of our lives each time slightly higher, gaining a different perspective at each turn of the same view, i.e. points A, B and C will all feel somewhat familiar – 'we had been there before' – but each time we complete a turn, we have an opportunity for a greater understanding or awareness of the same situation. We shall continue to meet the same problems and difficulties in our lives as we pursue our climbs – but on each occasion we have more information to comprehend the meaning and arrive at a resolution. Our age in years may not correspond to our psychological age, and the expression 'grown old before her time' or 'she will never grow up' reflects this awareness. We are often taxed with a responsibility beyond our means – there is no race to get to the top of the mountain and we may well have to wait and reflect on the 'view' we have available to us before moving on. Sometimes it may be necessary to retread our path so as to retrieve something we have mislaid before proceeding.

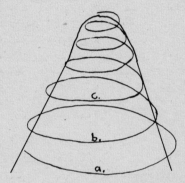

The Mountain of Life

Look at the diagram and make your own 'diagram', filling in the spaces with both your past experiences, achievements, as well as your future hopes. It is often possible to recognise an event which seemed to bring about a 'shift' between one stage and the next. These are often 'ritualised' in traditional societies by the building of a ceremony or feast. These ceremonies have been labelled 'rites of passage' and often help to foster the necessary circumstances for a further level of consciousness to be attained. If the rituals become empty and lose their meaning or are conducted with little or no 'awareness', then both individuals and societies may become stagnant unless they develop and create new 'rituals' which embody both meaning and mystery.

BODY	MIND	SPIRIT	RELATION-SHIP	ENVIRON-MENT
How does each *stage of your* *life relate to the* *categories?* *What do you* *see as the task* *for you?* Exercise Food Illness Health	Thoughts Feelings Ideas	Beliefs Values Experience	Family Friends Community Society	Plants Animals Air Water Earth Fire

OLD AGE
75+

RETIREMENT
65–75

PRE-RETIREMENT
55–65

MID-LIFE
45–55

MATURITY
35–45

SETTLING DOWN
25–35

YOUNG ADULT
18–25

ADOLESCENT
13–18

SCHOOL
0–13

THE 'MOUNTAIN' OF LIFE

Time management

Increasing awareness

Leave your watch behind one day a week. Notice how often you search for clocks to tell you the time. Gradually avoid looking for the 'external' clock and increase your sensitivity to your 'internal' clock.

Plan a weekend when you will follow your internal clock only. Eat when you feel like eating, sleep when you are tired and go to the lavatory not 'on time', but when your body says you need to.

Keep a diary for two days. Record everything you do, from the moment you wake up to when you go to sleep. Record the time you travel or read the newspaper. Record the time you wait for something to happen or watch television etc.

Finding the rhythm in your life

List all the major changes that have occurred to you since your earliest memories. Changes of school, job, partners, any illnesses, hospitalisations, operations. List any major goals or ambitions you have accomplished and any you have not. A creative way to do this is to draw a circle and put your current age somewhere along this circle, then fill the circle with your own ideas, hopes, fantasies of what may be in store for you.

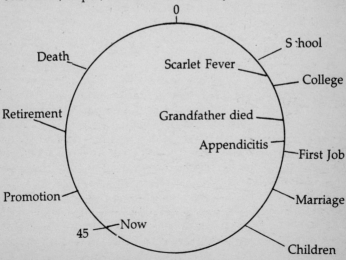

Anticipatory planning

The last exercise can be expanded to help you anticipate likely stressors in the future. Make a list of all the expected events in your life in:

    (1) The next week.
    (2) The next month.
    (3) The next year.
    (4) The next five years.

Include both those events you think will happen and those you would like to happen.

Creating time

The answer to finding time to do everything you have to do is a mixture of many things. Some of these ideas may help:

    (1) Plan and organise your timetable well ahead.
    (2) Make priorities of what has to be achieved.
    (3) Put off less urgent items.
    (4) Learn to say no.
    (5) Reduce the time you watch television.
    (6) Get up half-an-hour earlier.
    (7) Try and handle paperwork only once.
    (8) Take the telephone off the hook when you do not want to be disturbed.

Quiet time, quality time, quantity time

    (1) Give yourself 10 minutes to yourself every day. If you know you are going to be very busy and preoccupied with many decisions, pencil in an appointment with yourself. Learn to take control of time rather than have time take control of you.
    (2) Separate those tasks that require just a quantity of time to complete and are routine and mundane from those which require your full attention.

Transcending time

Once a month allow yourself at least three hours in which you have no tasks, no objectives, and let go of the time framework you normally exist in. Find a park, or a country lane, or a favourite place and spend intervals of meditation interspersed with intervals of focussing on your surroundings. Leave your watch behind!

13

HOW TO SEEK HELP

One of the major assumptions we have made in this book has been the question of responsibility. We have assumed that each individual is responsible for his or her own health – but responsible for what? Responsible for keeping fit, or preventing illness or responsible for treatment as well? We have also emphasised the importance of the environment we live in and the policies of conservation and preservation as they relate to our health. Surely as members of society we are also in part responsible for the way that society manages its affairs.

How far does this responsibility then go? One of the criticisms laid against the self-help, natural or holistic movement is that it blames the individual for his or her misfortunes, so that the patient has to cope not only with the illness but also with the guilt of knowing he is responsible for it. If there is little or no progress in treatment, then somehow he is doing something wrong. A further criticism is that it presumes an omnipotence – 'I can do anything if I want to' or 'I think positively and all will be well'.

A certain amount of individual responsibility is crucial to the holistic approach, but it includes being aware of one's limitations and the importance of seeking help from more knowledgeable and more competent people when appropriate. A holistic approach is not a 'do it yourself', 'I don't need anyone else' approach. It recognises the autonomy, strength and integrity of the individual and the power that comes from surrendering to the influence of others you trust, respect and love. Seeking help involves starting from within and working out to others.

Help from within

Prevention is better than cure both as practised by the individual and the doctor and *Health maintenance* and *disease prevention* are the first important forms of 'help' you can give yourself. The majority of exercises in this book aim to guide you into developing your own programme. Choose those that you enjoy and build slowly. Do not be hard on yourself if you 'fail' to keep your schedule, and allow yourself some room for change. Ensure you maintain an awareness of body-mind-spirit and work within your limitations.

Becoming ill or developing symptoms is part of our essential humanness and need not be seen as a 'fault' or 'sin'. The majority of imbalances or symptoms go away on their own if you provide the right environment. Indeed, over 75 per cent of all symptoms are never reported to a doctor or professional helper at all. But how do you decide whether a symptom is serious or not? A certain amount of *self-diagnosis* is essential and should be encouraged. Apart from the obvious emergency life-threatening symptoms these are some of the more important symptoms for which you should seek professional help as soon as possible.

Cough with blood or thick coloured phlegm
Chest pain
Headaches that recur frequently
Bleeding from anus, penis, vagina or mouth
Change in bowel habit over one month
Abdominal pain, especially if accompanied by diarrhoea
Pain on passing water
Lump in breast or elsewhere increasing in size
Unexplained loss of weight
Skin irritation or rash that persists
Skin mole that changes colour or bleeds easily
Ankle swelling that does not go away
Longstanding depression

The majority of symptoms that we get do not fall into this category and include the *physical* symptoms of headache, cold, slight cough, dizziness, nausea, generally feeling unwell, and the *mental* symptoms of tiredness, lassitude, depression, anxiety and irritability. These symptoms can be seen as the warning sign that something has gone wrong with our 'balance'. The symptoms should be seen not only as an unpleasant experience but also as an opportunity to explore *why* you are out of balance.

Ask yourself the question, 'What is this symptom trying to tell me?' Sometimes it is helpful to translate it into words – if you have a throbbing headache it might be translatable as 'I can't stand all this pressure around me' or tension in the back of the neck might mean 'I feel as if I have been strangled by all I have to do'. Giving your symptoms words may help you understand why you have developed them and point to ways in which you can moderate them. Some people find they can draw or paint their headaches or tiredness. We have already mentioned the use of a diary in which you keep all your thoughts and feelings and fantasies. This is yet another method to help you identify the meaning of your symptom or illness. It may not always be possible, or even desirable, to try to understand why you have got out of balance – all you may want to do is to restore yourself back to your normal state. Using Table I will help you to identify where the problem might be arising and what steps you may need to take.

Table I

Warning sign	Stressor	Stress response	Holistic response	DO IT YOURSELF		
	Job ? Relation- ships Food Environ- ment Memories Future work Money	Fight? Flight? Flow?	Breathing/ relaxation Meditation Exercise Food Visualisation Diary Time man- agement	Music Books Sleep Listen to tape Need help from outside	Walking Knitting Cooking Painting Mastur- bating Bath Tele- vision	? Tranquil- liser Herbal Teas Homoeo- pathic remedies
						Alcohol Tobacco Drugs

(1) **List your symptoms as 'warning signs' in column 1.**
  (a) separate those you have had for a long time from those that are new.

(2) **List your stressors, both internal and external.**
  - (a) Is the problem that you have too many?
  - (b) Are some stressors unchangeable (invalid relative, unemployment)?
  - (c) Do you have enough stressors?

(3) **For each stressor, list your stress response.**
  - (a) Is it the appropriate stress response?
  - (b) Would you wish to respond differently?
  - (c) Can you respond differently?

(4) **Go through the 'Holistic/Response' list and add any you have of your own.**
  - (a) Which one would be helpful to you at the moment?
  - (b) Are you tense, irritable, anxious,

or

  - (c) low, depressed and lethargic?
  - (d) Do you need to think clearly,

or

  - (e) Organise your timetable?
  - (f) Do you need to get rid of energy,

or

  - (g) Do you need comfort and looking after?
  - (h) Can you look after your own needs or do you need help from someone?
  - (i) Do you need to resort to alcohol, tobacco or drugs or can you do without?

(5) **A short cut and a simple way to help yourself is to use the diagram opposite.**

(1) Which quadrant describes your present state?
  - – High energy MIND
  - – High energy BODY
  - – Low energy MIND
  - – Low energy BODY

(2) What can you do to bring your current state back to the midline? You may find that if you are in a high energy or low energy *mind* state, you may need to do something with your *body*, e.g. physical exercise or breathing routine and vice versa.

(3) Remember the most effective 'stress managers' are those that have a wide range of 'holistic responses' available to them.

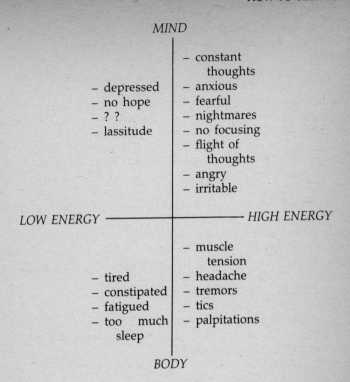

MIND

- constant
  thoughts
- depressed   - anxious
- no hope   - fearful
- ? ?   - nightmares
- lassitude   - no focusing
                  - flight of
                    thoughts
                  - angry
                  - irritable

LOW ENERGY ──────────────── HIGH ENERGY

                  - muscle
                    tension
- tired   - headache
- constipated   - tremors
- fatigued   - tics
- too much   - palpitations
  sleep

BODY

Seeking help from others

You've decided that your own resources are not sufficient and the difficulty or problem you face would be better dealt with by someone else; or perhaps you feel that you would like another person's viewpoint. Before we explore the professional sources of help, let us look at your own network. Again, it seems that the majority of us use our own families and friends as our first source of help. It is helpful to sort out in your own mind whether you are looking for special advice or just someone to listen to you. Choosing the person you seek help from may depend on what sort of help you need. You may prefer to seek out someone who knows nothing about you, or you may find yourself always going to your best friend. We all have a tendency to seek out

197

those who are most likely to agree with us and what we are really looking for is someone to support our position rather than give another opinion. Sometimes, when the issue is to do with a 'life decision' or important career choice, it is extremely helpful if we know someone 'wise'. Having 'three wise men or women' you can turn to on occasions is as important as having a first-aid box in the home. He or she may be your parent or a teacher, an employer who took a particular interest in you, a favourite uncle, a priest or, as the Irish call them, a 'soul-friend'. Developing an intimate circle of friends as well as a small group of 'wise counsellors' is an important step in accepting responsibility for your own health.

Other non-professional sources of help may include phone-in programmes, agony aunts, your local barman or barmaid. There has been an explosion of self-help groups and voluntary agencies and these are often run by people who may have experience of the same difficulty or problem you are having.

What do you want from a friend?
- a shoulder to cry on
- advice
- to be told what to do
- sympathy
- somebody to agree with you
- to be listened to
- to be distracted

Again, try and clarify in your own mind what it is you are seeking. A slightly more 'formal' way of seeking help but not one which is necessarily 'professional' or 'fee paying' is 'co-counselling'. This approach was developed in the 1950s and 1960s as a way of by-passing expensive psychotherapy and providing a model in which the relationship between the 'client' and 'therapist' is reversible, i.e. you take it in turn with your partner to be both the client and the therapist. Another feature of this form of counselling is that the 'client' remains in control and avoids the 'dependency', 'victim', 'child' role that may occur in more formal long-term psychotherapy. Co-counselling is a more sophisticated form of friendship in which a limited amount of training provides a major increase in skills and resources.

Professional help

*Sources of primary professional
care*
Non-fee paying
- Pharmacist
- General Practitioner
- Casualty
- Citizens Advice Bureau
- Social Services
- Drop-in Counselling Clinics
- Community Service Units
- Voluntary Agencies:
  - Mind
  - Age Concern
  - NSPCC
  - Community Health
    Council
  - Priest
Fee-paying
- Private Practitioners
  - Medical
  - Complementary
    Practitioners
  - Counsellor/
    Psychotherapist
- Marriage Guidance
  Counsellor
- Career Consultants

For the majority of people, the first professional person they will think of approaching is their general practitioner. This is, without doubt, one of the strengths of the National Health Service. Every individual has a right to a general practitioner in his own neighbourhood. In many countries where a strong general practitioner service does not exist, quite often the patient has to decide whether to seek a gastroenterologist or a cardiologist or a gynaecologist for him or herself. If he or she chooses the wrong specialist, it may be many investigations later, including unnecessary operations, before the 'mistake' is corrected. Developing a good relationship with your general practitioner is as much your responsibility as it is his or hers.

199

How to get the best out of your general practitioner

(a) Creating a good relationship requires time, commitment and involvement

If you see your GP infrequently, it may take a while to build up a relationship of trust. You can help by trying to see your own GP every time you need to, even if it may mean delaying an appointment for a few days. You are free to choose your GP and also free to change. The best recommendation is from other 'patients'. Ask around your pharmacist or health food store. Your local library or Community Health Council will keep a list of local practices. What sort of doctor do you want? A 'formal, business-like, competent scientist', a 'father-like figure – wise and slightly disorganised' or a 'friendly, non-authoritarian you-make-the-decisions' type?

It is a common observation that patients choose the sort of doctors they need, so don't be afraid to make your own conscious choice.

(b) Appointments, visits and second opinions

It is wise to have some understanding of practice policy regarding the above 'practicalities'. If you feel your problem may require slightly longer time, ask, if necessary, by letter, for a longer appointment. Most practices operate a policy of visiting their own patients during daylight hours and having a rota or emergency back-up system at night. Requests for visits need to be rung in as early as possible and it does no harm to make sure you get on with the receptionists (a bunch of flowers or gifts at Christmas are far more appropriately given to the reception staff than to the doctor). Asking your doctor for a second opinion is your right and should be used more often than is done. Nevertheless, it puts an onus on you to be clear as to why you need a second opinion. Spend a little time clarifying in your own mind what you would like from your doctor before you see him. Let him know if there are underlying personal stresses which may be affecting your physical health – remember it is *your* body and *your* mind.

Other 'first-hand' sources of professional help are listed in Table 0 and for many people provide not only a refuge in time of crisis but a supportive framework over a longer period of time.

One group to which the public appears to be turning to more frequently is the complementary or 'alternative' practitioner who mostly operates on a fee-paying basis. There is an increasing confusion as to which 'alternative' therapy should be sought for which condition. Before embarking on a brief guide, it is helpful to explore why it is that people turn to alternative medicine. Some of the reasons may appear 'health-promoting', others are often not. Which reasons apply to you?

'Good reason'	'Bad reason'
Want more time with practitioner	
Think therapy will help	Looking for 'magical' solution
Need to be under guidance of 'therapist'	Do not want to explore psychological area
Prefer 'holistic' approach	
Want to be more involved in own therapy	

One of the more disheartening trends is to see patients who have sought me out to 'try some of your holistic tablets'. They have usually tried homoeopathy, acupuncture, herbalism, etc., and shop around hoping to avoid looking at their own responsibility. The search for a 'magic bullet' has been replaced by a search for a 'magical therapy'.

Nevertheless, a welcome change has occurred amongst the medical profession in recent years and there is now a greater acceptance of the efficacy of alternative therapies. We provide below a brief guide to the major therapies – not all have adequate educational and ethical regulation support and it is important to ask for information from some of the 'umbrella' organisations that keep registers and lists of recognised groups.

Major complementary therapies

There are five major complementary therapies which offer good training and regulatory bodies with ethical and clinical guidelines:

(1) Acupuncture

This is an approach to treatment based on the Chinese model of health and disease. In this model, it is felt that in addition to a circulatory and nervous system, energy flows in channels called meridians and disease occurs where the energy flow is blocked for whatever reason. Needles are placed in different parts of the body and help to 'unblock' energy channels. The placing of needles is only one aspect of acupuncture and a physician trained in traditional Chinese medicines will take a very long time to arrive at his 'diagnosis' and will pay particular attention to diet, emotional and environmental factors. In Britain there are two 'schools' of acupuncture practice. One is based on the traditional Chinese approach, is practised mostly by non-doctors and generally accepts a wide range of problems. The second school is practised by doctors and is based much more on a western model of disease. Acupuncture (the placing of needles) is seen as an additional 'treatment' and is most commonly used for muscular and arthritic conditions – the relief of pain and occasionally for anaesthesia. There is an unfortunate division between these two schools and it can be problematic for the patient to know where to go to seek help.

(2) Osteopathy

This is a well-accepted approach for the treatment of many muscular, skeletal and arthritic conditions. The practitioners receive a perfectly good training and treat these conditions with a mixture of massage, manipulation and exercise retraining and postural advice. Quite often a low back pain not managed by conventional medical treatment (drugs, rest or surgery) has been dramatically helped by the use of osteopathic techniques. Some osteopaths will expand their clinical practice to include more general conditions, e.g. asthma, migraine, etc.

(3) Chiropractic

This is very similar to osteopathy but much less available in the UK. The difference has more to do with the type of manipulative technique used and the range of conditions treated.

(4) Herbal medicine

There is a long tradition of using herbs for the treatment of medical conditions – indeed, many of our most effective drugs are derived from medical herbs (Digitalis – Foxglove). Herbalists are trained in anatomy, physiology and diagnosis much like most doctors, but use herbs instead of drugs for their therapies. Herbalists will treat the whole gamut of medical conditions, although they will be quite happy to refer back to the doctor those conditions which are better treated by conventional means.

(5) Homoeopathy

This branch of complementary medicine has a long and traditional history in Britain, having been the preferred approach to treatment amongst many members of the Royal Family. The majority of homoeopaths are doctors who have been trained in a conventional manner. Homoeopathy is a system of therapeutics (treatment) using 'remedies' rather than drugs. These remedies contain minute levels of extracts which have no 'chemical effect' on the body. Homoeopaths believe remedies work as a result of the fundamental principle of homoeopathy that 'like cures like'. By this is meant that instead of suppressing or destroying a symptom or infection (as modern drugs do), cure is achieved by stimulating the body's own healing powers. This is done by giving a remedy which, in much greater doses, would *produce* the actual symptom the patient is complaining about.

There is no doubt that homoeopathy is a safe method of treatment and that in several conditions it appears to have a dramatic effect. Conventional doctors are still unconvinced that it has a part to play in the treatment of disease and there has been little objective evidence to indicate that homoeopathy is effective in acute and chronic disease states. Nevertheless, for many of the minor to moderately severe non-life-threatening conditions, homoeopathy is a safe and effective therapy. It must be pointed out that many of these conditions are self-limiting and would probably improve whatever therapy was used.

Unlike conventional medicine, there is no 'general practitioner' of complementary therapies, and it is difficult to decide which therapy to seek out. Many more GPs are now knowledgeable and sympathetic towards complementary therapies and it is as well to discuss your request first with him or her. The British Holistic Medical Association (medical, complementary and lay membership) operates an information and advice service, and if in doubt you can seek its advice.

14

THE HOLISTIC APPROACH – A SEARCH FOR MEANING

Is it possible in this last chapter to bring together all the different elements described in the previous chapters? What sort of whole can be made from all the different parts? In many ways this has been the central theme of the book – that searching for the whole or trying to make sense of the disparate experiences in our lives is the struggle and purpose for all of us. At times of financial hardship or emotional turmoil or physical distress, it may appear that the part of us which is unbalanced is all that we need to concern ourselves with, or indeed are able to concern ourselves with. We get drawn into the *part* and let go of the *whole*, incomplete, foggy and indeterminate as it is. It is as if we are all engaged in a giant jigsaw puzzle but have no clear view of what the whole picture looks like. We get taken up by a small part of the picture or even just a small piece of the jigsaw itself and spend all our energies in identifying with or attempting to resolve that portion of the jigsaw.

Trying to complete a jigsaw puzzle without access to the complete picture is not impossible, but it is much easier if you have the picture by you. Similarly, trying to find your way from point A to point B without a map or guide is possible and you may be fortunate to have an unerring sense of direction – or you quite rightly enjoy the pleasure and sense of fun that results from exploring with no fixed end in sight and no point B to get to. The world's great religions, Christianity, Buddhism, Judaism, Islam, have all set out to provide maps of the human condition and described ways of getting from point A to point B. Through their priests, rabbis, imams and swamis, they have provided guides and leaders to take us from 'darkness to light' or from the 'unreal to the real'. Each of the great religions will point to special individuals – Christ, Krishna, Buddha, Mohammed, Moses – who in their view are examples of the 'whole picture' or point B. In the great books – the Bible, Koran, Bagavad Gita – there are chapters on ways of reaching point B and exercises describing the preparation that is necessary before embarking on that journey.

The secular version of this search is evidenced by the numerous 'self-help' books and 'How to . . .' guides that are a feature of many modern bookstores. The principal danger of making the 'final picture' or point B or a 'beautiful body' or a 'quiet mind' as the goal of the journey or search is that one may lose sight of 'the way'. By this I mean that *the way of travelling is the picture, is point B*. If we lose sight of that then we run the risk of confusing 'part' of the picture with the whole. Much of the persecution occurring under the name of religion, the major religious wars, the enmity between even different sects of Christianity, is the result of people disagreeing and fighting over which point B is the correct one. Imagine a group of people trying to complete a jigsaw puzzle, each having a different idea of what the final picture should look like and each determined to prove that his 'vision' is the right one. *But then even the way of travelling may also be different*. Some of us may like the challenge of the short but difficult route – others may prefer the circuitous, scenic road, stopping frequently to enjoy the view. Some may prefer to travel alone, whilst others will join a group and tread the road to 'Canterbury' as a 'band of pilgrims'.

'How confusing – first you say there is no agreed final picture and now you say there is no agreed common path!' No wonder so few people complete the jigsaw, so many give up and lead lives of quiet desperation, or that squabbles, quarrels, fights and wars are so prevalent. What hope is there for the individual struggling to keep a balance between his inner confusion and outer chaos. But wait, it may be this urge, this drive to keep struggling that will provide the clue. It is this urge or drive to 'wholeness' that some will call the 'spirit' of man and woman. The spirit of man has been referred to tangentially throughout this book, although we have not devoted a chapter to it. It is the energy, driving force, vitality, 'life force', 'something beyond ourselves' that will provide us with inspiration, belief, conviction. When our body and mind is enthused with a sense of 'the spirit', then we may feel 'at one', 'a sense of harmony', 'a feeling of peace', a 'knowing' that is from somewhere within and not an intellectual knowing.

What can be said from comparing the 'great books' and the

teachings of the 'great souls' is that their descriptions of 'the spirit', even though they call it by different names, are remarkably similar. Down through the centuries poets, mystics, scientists have struggled to describe in words that which is beyond words. But what 'that' is seems crucial to this book, for it may help to link the parts together. The parts (separate chapters) on their own may indeed be helpful and may have helped you identify separate parts of your own jigsaw, but how do you bring the separate parts together? Just to remind you (BODY - MIND-BREATH-DIET-EXERCISE-MEDITATION-RELATION-SHIPS - SEX - WORK - ENVIRONMENT - TIME). I propose we call the glue that binds these parts together in a harmonious whole – 'spirit' or holism, or, if you prefer, any of the other words that have been used (Table 0).

Other words for Spirit	
Soul	Tao
Consciousness	Breath of life
Higher self	Energy
'It'	Holism
Élan vital	Prana
Chi	

It is important to stress at this point that for the moment I am separating the word 'spirit' from any religious connotation but looking at it from the point of view of 'that which binds the parts together and makes the whole greater than the sum of the parts'.

The holistic approach and the spiritual path

Let us draw together certain aspects of the holistic approach which have been mentioned from time to time in the previous chapters and examine how they not only provide the links that bind the parts but also the 'whole' that is made up of the parts.

Awareness
Being fully aware is being fully alive, and being fully alive is being enthused with spirit. Whether you jog daily, eat only organic food, meditate for one hour a day or have regular check-

ups, the central important question is how aware you are of your own experience. How aware of the external environment coming in through your senses (sight, sound, smells etc.), and how aware of your internal environment (thoughts, fantasies, feelings). Another word for awareness is consciousness. How conscious are you of your own self, with a small 's', and Self with a capital 'S'? The amount of awareness you are able to bring to whatever activity you perform, from washing-up to walking to the bus, to paying your bills, to suffering with a headache, will help to enhance, encourage and cultivate your spirit. This may explain why so many people who neither jog nor meditate nor worry about their diet are able to lead such seemingly tranquil, peaceful and fulfilled lives. Another way to translate awareness is the invocation 'Be here now'. Throughout this book, in all the exercises we have described, we have focussed on the awareness you bring to that exercise and in the section on meditation we have indicated ways in which you can begin to attain some mastery over your attention, awareness and consciousness.

Responsibility

To achieve awareness, you have to begin to take responsibility for doing so yourself. This has been another of the central themes passing through this book. The responsibility you take is not the 'I can do it all myself', 'I don't need anyone else' variety, it is the responsibility to be fully aware – fully aware of your strengths as well as your weaknesses, fully aware of your own capacity to heal yourself as well as your own incapacity to do so. Taking responsibility for yourself is not the same as saying you should feel guilty if your life is in a mess or your health is not perfect. Taking responsibility does mean, though, choosing your own path in life whether it is the 'short cut' or the meandering lane. It does mean choosing whether to accept the 'whole picture' as described by others or searching for your own 'whole picture'. Taking responsibility for yourself involves you in becoming aware of yourself as well as others, for part of yourself is in others.

Interconnectedness

St Augustine's definition of a sin was the 'turning away from the universal whole to the individual part'. Increasing our awareness and taking responsibility for ourselves leads us to the understanding of how the parts of our selves and our lives are connected. We have shown in various chapters how the body is linked to the mind and vice versa. All disease is psychosomatic in that both body and mind are involved. We have seen that not only is our body made up of what we eat but that the process of eating and breathing connects us to the world of nature, the animals and plants as well as the air, sea and earth. We do not live in a universe where we are here and everything else is out there.

This notion of subject (you) and object (the world) as being separate and distinct is no longer tenable. Modern science through quantum physics has shown how what we observe and measure is affected by the consciousness (awareness) we bring to the observation and measurement. We live in a participatory world and each of us is connected in some way or another to everyone else. Becoming aware of this connectedness will ensure, as so many of the good books say, that you 'look after your neighbour as yourself', for in looking after your 'neighbour', be it within your marriage, at your work place, in your social set, you will also be looking after yourself. Hans Selye, who found many of his neighbours difficult to love, translated this precept into what he called 'selfish altruism' and used the invocation, 'Earn thy neighbour's love', which put the onus on his neighbours to love him rather than the other way round!

Balance

Bringing the last three dimensions to the foreground will entail the difficult task of finding the right balance between the opposing forces present in one's life. How do I choose between the needs of my body and those of my mind? How do I find the balance between the need to be alone and separate and the need to be with others and in a group? How do I find the balance between working and playing, sadness and joy, the needs of my family and my own individual needs? We indicated in Chapter 9 how our reality is basically shaped by the series of polarities or opposites, and how when we use such words as happy, active, healthy, fulfilled, we also demonstrate our notions of the opposite – unhappy, passive, ill-health, unfulfilled. It can be said that our education and culture has aided in developing the belief, pursuing the notion, and celebrating the illusion that we can have one side of this equation without the other. There can be no rich persons if there are no poor, there can be no good people if there are no bad people.

This illusion of the one-sided nature of the human condition is equally prevalent in the notion of health and illness. The word 'health' comes from the same stem as the word 'wholeness', the Greek *holos*. Wholeness implies both the state of illness and the absence of illness. Someone who has no illness but little or no awareness is far less whole (healthy) than someone who is suffering from cancer or arthritis and is fully aware of the experience of being 'ill'. Finding the right balance, or, as the Buddhists would say 'the middle way', involves first reclaiming the *projected other half of the polarity* (see Chapter 9), finding the weak side of ourselves if we see ourselves as strong, or the feminine side if we see ourselves as masculine, the health side if we see ourselves as ill, etc. It involves seeing our lives as having both a spring and a summer as well as an autumn and winter (Chapter 12) and finally, involves us in developing the stance of non-attachment.

Non-attachment

Finding a balance between two opposing forces does not mean finding a compromise and although it may entail that, non-attachment does not imply detachment or indifference. Non-attachment incolves a tolerant acceptance or benevolent understanding of two opposing tensions: it does not mean a painful acquiescence or a cynical perspective. Developing non-attachment involves one in letting go of both the pleasure and the pain, the rewards of success as well as the disappointments of failure. This does not mean that emotions are avoided and suppressed, they are fully felt in the here and now but equally they are let go of as the moment changes.

People who have developed the art of non-attachment are truly spontaneous, 'child-like' in their responses, expressing both anger and joy but having 'no memory or desire'. Jung described this state as 'the art of letting things happen': 'Action through non-action, letting go of oneself as taught by Meister Eckhart became for me the key that opens the door to the way . . . this is an art about which most people know nothing. Consciousness is forever interfering. It would be simple enough if only simplicity were not the most difficult of all things.' How can we develop the art of non-attachment? How can we avoid identifying ourselves with one aspect of the polarity – 'I want to be good', 'I want to be happy', 'I want to be healthy', 'I want to be rich', etc.? Non-attachment involves letting go of all addictions and all dependencies. Not just addiction to tobacco or alcohol or chocolate cakes or sex, but addiction to desire to be healthy or be loved or be 'at peace'. For whilst we are attached to and dependent on the need to 'achieve success' or 'be peaceful', then we shall continue to experience the one-sidedness of the polarity to which we are addicted.

When we do not get our desire or have it taken away, then we shall experience all the distress and pain of withdrawal symptoms. Non-attachment does not mean no-action but it does mean 'not being attached to the fruits of your action'. Non-attachment develops through an increased awareness and a transcending of the polarities, and an increased awareness of the complementary nature of the polarities arises out of the state of non-attachment. Non-attachment leads to greater awareness and a greater awareness leads to non-attachment. This non-attachment allows us to find the balance between the polarities of our lives.

Grace of God – surrendering to the whole
In this journey towards wholeness, we shall all arrive at a point in our lives when we feel stuck, either in a physical illness or an external calamity or psychological cul-de sac. Howevec much we struggle to find a solution, search for a meaning, develop a non-attached attitude, we will feel caught by the unmitigating hold of our own desires, memories, actions and egos. Meditate as we will, jog till the cows come home, breathe till you are relaxed, out of your mind, the distress, the attachment, the dis-ease returns. You seek help as outlined in Chapter 13, you visit your 'wise men' or lie on a psychiatrist's couch for a few years, take a host of vitamin tablets or explore acupuncture, but still that feeling of emptiness, disjointedness or alienation persists. The philosophy of the holistic approach suggests not only that the whole is greater than the sum of the parts, but that the whole is contained in each smallest part: remember Blake – 'To see a world in a grain of sand'.

Letting go of our small part and surrendering to the greater whole is what Christians would say is being touched by the Grace of God. No one can guarantee that it will happen, no scientific measuring instrument can attest to its occurrence, yet it is a belief in all the great religions, especially the Judaeo-

211

Christian-Muslim traditions. The ultimate Whole or God is seen as transcending and 'ruling over' the universe, and man is seen as but an infinitesimally small part of that universe. None the less the invocation is to 'have faith and all shall be revealed'. Even in the eastern religions, Buddhism, Hinduism, Jainism, where the concept of the ultimate reality is that it resides in each one of us and is immanent rather than transcendent, the issue of 'surrendering' is crucial to the relationship between the small self and the big Self.

Many of our greatest saints and mystics call this point 'the dark night of the soul', where all that is possible is having faith in the presence of the absolute, the totality, God. For many, this faith, some would say 'blind faith', is transferred on to human beings, the preacher or guru or doctor. This surrendering can often be a way of avoiding responsibility – 'You tell me what to do, doctor/priest/teacher/wise man, and I will do it'. True surrender to the power of Grace or the ultimate comes after true responsibility not before, but the unwillingness to let go of responsibility and surrender to the Greater Whole will perpetuate the attachment to the 'part'.

Forgiveness

This last element of the holistic approach may appear slightly out of place and it has not been a prominent feature in earlier chapters. Nevertheless, it seems important to include it as it is so necessary for progress to be made. In our search for wholeness, we shall inevitably stumble, fail, slip backwards, descend into un-consciousness and generally make a mess of things. We shall eat the wrong food, forget to breathe properly, indulge in heavy drinking, upset our family and friends and avoid our responsibilities. We shall break our own rules, fail to meet our own standards and forget our own good intentions.

Not only that, we shall constantly be in the company of other human beings who are just the same. They will fail to meet our expectations, disappoint us, let us down and generally make our lives more difficult. Our wives/husbands will stop loving us, fail to support us in our time of need and seem determined to pursue their own selfish goals. Our children will not grow up to be what we would like them to be, they will reject our values, discard their heritage and develop their own separate and, at times, alien lifestyles. On this journey we shall meet parents, teachers, doctors, priests and other guides who will let us down and turn out to be yet more false prophets. Our beliefs and values will at times become a 'heap of broken images' and it will appear as if we are surrounded by fools, liars and knaves.

Without the willingness and capacity to forgive these many disappointments and disillusionments, we will be forever stuck in the imperfectness of the 'part'. Forgiveness starts with the forgiveness we give to ourselves and arises out of the awareness of the incompleteness of the 'part' that we identify with, whether it be our physique, or our intelligence or our status and wealth. Forgiveness of others for their shortcomings follows once we have accepted our shortcomings. True forgiveness implies first an awareness of the weak/damaged/failed/arrogant/conceited/unfinished part and then a letting go of this part so that the search for wholeness can be allowed to continue.

Death and dying

A book on holistic living could not omit the subject of death and some would say we should have started with our attitudes towards death. For these attitudes determine, in large part, the way we live. In an uncertain and chaotic world, the only certainty is the inevitability of our own death. Yet as a culture, we avoid talking about it, it is thought morbid to dwell on it. A major part of our health care system is devoted to a battle with death. Doctors and nurses consider themselves to have failed if a patient dies. A vast technology has arisen to prolong life at whatever cost and the very process of dying has been medicalised. Fewer and fewer people die at home – death is no longer an event that a small child will witness as part of the cycle of life. In hospital, the culture is one of denial, amongst the medical profession as well as relatives and patients – 'Don't tell him, doctor, he will give up hope', 'It is cruel to tell him he is going to die' are common statements.

The human feelings surrounding death are banished with admonitions against showing emotions – 'It will only upset you' – to the prescription of tranquillisers, barbiturates and other sedatives. In many cases what people are frightened of is not death itself, but the process of dying. The fear is in part due to the concern over 'pain' or 'being a burden', but more often than not it is the fear of having to cope with the feelings surrounding a dying person. All these feelings have been well described by Elisabeth Kubler-Ross, and her followers have done much to ensure that the subject of death has come out from behind the closet. Ross describes the five states that she observed many terminally ill people go through:

(a) Denial
People do not 'hear' or do not wish to hear their prognosis, they put on a brave face and both relatives and medical personnel collude with this denial as it makes their task that much easier.

(b) Anger
'Why me?', or anger at the medical profession for not making the right diagnosis in time and giving the wrong treatment. The anger can be directed at relatives or nurses or at themselves for failing to have a check-up etc.

(c) Bargaining
'How long do I have to live? If I am good/take the tablets/keep to the diet/will I have longer?' In this stage, the patient is most co-operative and will do almost anything to ward off death, even agreeing to heroic surgery, and visiting unconventional healers.

(d) Depression
The inevitability of their death finally is faced and with it comes the realisation of loss of loved ones, loss of material possessions and loss of life. The person feels abandoned, rejected and alone.

(e) Acceptance
For those who reach this final stage, there arrives a state of peace and tranquillity. They regain their spontaneity and joy and live for the now, the moment they exist. Even though they may be weak, in pain or discomfort, they are fully alive and could be said to be at their healthiest.

It is unfortunate that very few people reach the stage of acceptance before their death. We have had no preparation for this moment. Indeed our major efforts have gone towards warding it off and denying its possibility. These attitudes are shaped by our education, culture and religious beliefs. Do we believe in an after-life? Is there really a heaven and hell? Will we really be called to judgment for our misdemeanours? The Judaeo-Christian tradition, with its emphasis on punishment and redemption, has helped to shape these attitudes and death has become something to be frightened of. The eastern religions place a different emphasis on death, seeing it no more and no less than what it is – the natural and inevitable culmination of life. They see life as the preparation for death and feel only able to say whether a man's life has been successful or not after they have witnessed his mode of dying. This attitude is also found amongst the Stoics, and Leonardo da Vinci wrote, 'Just as a day well spent brings happy sleep, so a life well spent brings happy death'.

A holistic approach to living involves having a holistic approach to your own death. It involves seeing attachment to life much as one would see attachment to other habits. Yes, there to be enjoyed, but there also to be released lest the habit become an addiction from which withdrawal would produce the pain and torment so evident in people's lives. Thus the holistic approach involves one in the search for meaning, but this meaning may and will shift from day to day, or even hour by hour. The same set of facts will appear differently on a different day or if you are in a different mood. Allowing for multiple and different levels of meaning will ensure that you do not confuse facts with truth. Having to face these multiple levels of meaning will force you into making choices. The choices you make will be evidence of your own free-will and will be the steps you lay down for your own journey through life. As you travel along that journey, in the pursuit of the meaning to your life, a holistic approach will ensure that your pursuit of your truth will be tinged with the awareness of the importance of the present moment – the ephemeral nature of your life and the inevitability of your death.

Organisations and associations

GENERAL ORGANISATIONS

BRITISH HOLISTIC MEDICAL ASSOCIATION
179 Gloucester Place, London NW1 6DX
01–262 5299/402 2768

information on holistic and complementary medicine;
educational activities; self-help cassettes, reading lists, leaflets;
newsletters and journal; membership open to the public

COLLEGE OF HEALTH
18 Victoria Park Square, London E2 9BR
01–980 6263
consumer organisation for NHS patients; interest in
complementary medicine; publications; journal;
membership open to the public

COUNCIL FOR COMPLEMENTARY AND
ALTERNATIVE MEDICINE
Suite 1, 19a Cavendish Square, London W1M 9AD
01–409 1440
concerned with standardisation of training, practice, code of
ethics and legislation within the professional associations

INSTITUTE FOR COMPLEMENTARY MEDICINE
21 Portland Place, London W1N 3AP
01–636 9543
information on complementary medicine; newsletter and
journal; membership open to the public

RESEARCH COUNCIL FOR COMPLEMENTARY
MEDICINE
Suite 1, 19a Cavendish Square, London W1M 9AD
01–493 6930
promotes and co-ordinates research; newsletter and journal

PROFESSIONAL ASSOCIATIONS

Acupuncture

BRITISH ACUPUNCTURE ASSOCIATION

34 Alderney Street
London SW1V 4EU
01–834 3353/1012

INTERNATIONAL REGISTER OF ORIENTAL MEDICINE

Green Hedges House, Green Hedges Avenue
East Grinstead, Sussex RH19 1DZ
0342 28567

TRADITIONAL ACUPUNCTURE SOCIETY

11 Grange Park
Stratford upon Avon, Warks CV37 6XH
0789 298798

Chiropractic

BRITISH CHIROPRACTORS' ASSOCIATION

5 First Avenue
Chelmsford, Essex CM1 1RX
0245 353078

Homoeopathy

BRITISH HOMOEOPATHIC ASSOCIATION

27a Devonshire Street
London W1N 1RJ
01–935 2163

SOCIETY OF HOMOEOPATHS

101 Sebastian Avenue
Shenfield
Brentwood, Essex CM15 8PP

Medical Herbalism

NATIONAL INSTITUTE OF MEDICAL HERBALISTS

148 Forest Road
Tunbridge Wells, Kent TN2 5EY
0892 30400

Osteopathy

BRITISH AND EUROPEAN OSTEOPATHIC ASSOCIATION

42–45 Broad Street
London EC2M 1QY
0233 31530

BRITISH NATUROPATHIC AND OSTEOPATHIC ASSOCIATION

Frazer House, 6 Netherhall Gardens
London NW3 5RR
01–435 8728

BRITISH OSTEOPATHIC ASSOCIATION

8–10 Boston Place
London NW1 6QH
01–262 5250

217

GENERAL COUNCIL AND REGISTER OF OSTEOPATHS
1–4 Suffolk Street
London SW1Y 4HG
01–839 2060

Each of these organisations will identify a local practitioner on request. Many of the registers will be available in public libraries.

ORGANISATIONS GIVING SERVICES AND HELP

Advisory Services to Patients
ARTHRITIS CARE
6 Grosvenor Crescent
London SW1X 7ER
01–235 0902
   information and advisory service; regional groups

BACUP (British Association for Cancer United Patients and their Families)
121–123 Charterhouse Street
London EC1M 6AA
01–608 1661
   information and advisory service, run by a team of doctors

CANCER LINK
46a Pentonville Road
London N1 9HF
01–833 2451
   one of many support groups in this field; regional groups

Counselling Services
CRUSE
Cruse House, 126 Sheen Road
Richmond, Surrey TW9 1UR
01–940 4818/9047
   bereavement counselling

NATIONAL MARRIAGE GUIDANCE COUNCIL
Herbert Gray College
Little Church Street
Rugby, Warks CV21 3AP
0788 73241

TAVISTOCK CLINIC
120 Belsize Lane
London NW3 5BA
01–435 7111

WESTMINSTER PASTORAL FOUNDATION
23 Kensington Square
London W8 5HN
01–937 6956

(For details of these and other agencies, consult *A referral directory of counselling agencies and organisations* listed below)

Diet and Nutrition
BRITISH SOCIETY FOR NUTRITIONAL MEDICINE
Information Officer: Dr Alan Stewart
5 Somerhill Road
Hove, East Sussex BN3 1RP
0273 722003
  name(s) of nearest nutritionist available on request

VEGETARIAN SOCIETY UK LTD
53 Marloes Road
London W8 6LA
01–937 7739/1714
  holds meetings and demonstrations; journal and other publications

Ecology
BRITISH SOCIETY FOR ALLERGY AND ENVIRONMENTAL STUDIES
Mrs Ina Mansell
'Acorns', Romsey Road
Cadman, Southampton SO4 2NN
0703 812124
  name(s) of local ecology practitioner available on request by a doctor only

FRIENDS OF THE EARTH
377 City Road
London EC1V 1NA
01–837 0731
  promotes rational use of natural resources

Exercise, Aerobics
AEROBIC AND FITNESS ASSOCIATION
29 Hursley Road
Chandlers Ford
Eastleigh, Hants SO5 2FS
04215 3084
  name(s) of a local teacher available on request

ASSET (National Association for Health and Exercise Teachers)
East Cottage Studios
Ashenden
Bayford, Herts SG13 8PZ
0865 736066
  name(s) of a local teacher available on request

BRITISH T'AI CHI CHUAN ASSOCIATION
7 Upper Wimpole Street
London W1M 7TD
01–935 8444
  name(s) of local teacher available on request

219

KEEP FIT ASSOCIATION

16 Upper Woburn Place
London WC1H 0QG
01–388 0828
> name of local secretary
> available on request;
> for details of local groups
> and classes, consult your
> public library

Psychology

INSTITUTE OF PSYCHOSYNTHESIS

1 Cambridge Gate
Regents Park, London NW1
4JN
01–486 2588
> short courses for the
> layman on integration of
> transpersonal and personal
> psychology; name(s) of a
> local counsellor available on
> request

INSTITUTE OF TRANSACTIONAL ANALYSIS

BM Box 4104, 27a Old
Gloucester Street
London WC1 3XX
01–404 5011
> short courses and
> workshops for the layman;
> name(s) of local therapist
> available on request

Relaxation, Stress Control

HEALTH EDUCATION COUNCIL

Look After Yourself Project
Christchurch College
Canterbury, Kent CT1 1QU
0227 455564
> nationwide courses on
> healthy living, including
> stress control and relaxation
> techniques; name of local
> co-ordinator available on
> request

STRESS FOUNDATION

Cedar House
Yalding, Kent ME18 6JD
0622 814431
> publications and self-help
> leaflets available

Yoga, Meditation

BRITISH SCHOOL OF YOGA

24 Osney Crescent
Paignton, Devon TQ4 5EY
0803 552090
> name(s) of local teacher
> available on request

BUDDHIST SOCIETY

58 Eccleston Square
London SW1 1PH
01–834 5858
> details of local group
> available on request

FURTHER READING

GENERAL

FULDER, Stephen *The handbook of complementary medicine*. Coronet Books, 1984

INGLIS, Brian and WEST, Ruth *The alternative health guide*. Michael Joseph, 1983

STANWAY, Andrew *Alternative medicine: a guide to natural therapies*. Penguin, 1982

DIRECTORIES

Charities digest. Published annually by Family Welfare Association, 501–505 Kingsland Road, London E8 4AU

Help! I need somebody: a guide to national associations for people in need, compiled by Sally Knight. 3rd edition. Published by Kimpton. 1980.

A referral directory of counselling agencies and organisations, edited by Anthony Clayton. Published by British Association for Counselling, 37a Sheep Street, Rugby, Warks. 1984.

Self-help and the patient: a directory of national organisations concerned with various diseases and handicaps. Published by Patients' Association, Room 33, 18 Charing Cross Road, London W2 0HR. 1984.

Someone to talk to directory 1985: a directory of self-help and community support agencies – national and local – in the UK and Republic of Ireland. Published by Routledge & Kegan Paul, for the Mental Health Foundation. 1985
(Most of these directories will be available in public libraries)

JOURNALS

HERE'S HEALTH Monthly
Argus Health Publications
30 Station Approach
West Byfleet, Surrey KT14 6NF

HOLISTIC HEALTH Quarterly
British Holistic Medical Association
179 Gloucester Place
London NW1 6DX
  available to members only

HOLISTIC MEDICINE Quarterly
British Holistic Medical Association
179 Gloucester Place
London NW1 6DX
  aimed primarily at the professional practitioner

JOURNAL OF ALTERNATIVE MEDICINE Monthly
Argus Health Publications
30 Station Approach
West Byfleet, Surrey KT14 6NF
  aimed primarily at the professional practitioner; available on
  subscription only

NEW HEALTH Monthly
Haymarket Publishing Ltd
38–42 Hampton Road
Teddington, Middx TW11 0JE

RECOMMENDED READING ON SPECIAL TOPICS

Chapter 1

CAPRA, Fritjof *The Tao of physics*. Fontana/Collins, 1975
— — *The turning point: science, society and the rising culture.*
Wildwood House, 1982.
ILLICH, Ivan *Limits to medicine: medical nemesis, the expropriation of health.* Boyars, 1976 (Penguin 1977, paper)
McKEOWN, Thomas *The role of medicine: dream, mirage or nemesis?* Blackwell, 1979
SELYE, Hans *Stress without distress.* New ed. Hodder & Stoughton, 1977
SHAH, Idries *Nasrudin: exploits of the incomparable Mulla Nasrudin.* New ed. Octagon Press, 1983

Chapter 2

SAGAN, Carl *The dragon of Eden: speculations on the evolution of human intelligence.* New ed. Hodder & Stoughton, 1979
SELYE, Hans *The stress of life.* 2nd ed. McGraw-Hill, 1978
TOFFLER, Alvin *Future shock.* New ed. Pan, 1973

Chapter 3

BENSON, Herbert *The relaxation response.* Collins, 1975
LAMBLEY, Peter *Insomnia and other sleeping problems.* Sphere, 1983
MADDERS, Jane *Stress and relaxation: self-help ways to cope with stress and relieve nervous tension, ulcers, insomnia, migraine and high blood pressure.* 3rd ed. Dunitz, 1981 (Positive health guides series)
NUERNBERGER, Phil *Freedom from stress.* Himalayan International Institute, 1981
TYRER, Peter *How to sleep better.* Sheldon Press, 1978

Chapter 4

BUPA manual of fitness and well-being. Macdonald, 1985
COOPER, Kenneth *Aerobics.* Bantam, 1968
— — and COOPER, Mildred *Aerobics for women.* Bantam, 1973
O'BRIEN, Justin *Running and breathing.* CSA Press, 1983
WICKS, *Guide to exercise.* Heart Foundation of Australia, 1982

Chapter 5

BALLENTINE, Rudolph *Diet and nutrition: a holistic approach.* Himalayan International Institute, 1978

HALL, Ross Hume *Food for nought: the decline in nutrition.* Vintage, 1976

HANSSEN, Maurice *E for additives: the complete 'E' number guides.* Thorsons, 1984

KIRSCHMANN, John D *Nutritional almanac.* Rev ed. McGraw-Hill, 1985

PLESHETTE, Janet *Health on your plate.* Hamlyn, 1983

POLUNIN, Miriam *The right way to eat: to feel good or even better.* Dent, 2nd ed. 1986.

Chapter 6

BLAKEMORE, Colin *Mechanics of the mind: BBC Reith lectures.* Cambridge University Press, 1977

RUSSELL, Peter *The brain book: know your own mind and how to use it.* New ed. Routledge & Kegan Paul, 1980

SCHUTZ, William *Profound simplicity.* Turnstone Press, 1979

Chapter 7

BLAKESLEE, Thomas R *The right brain.* Macmillan, 1980

DAVIS, Martha and others *Relaxation and stress reduction workbook.* New Harbinger Publications, 1980

GAWAIN, Shakli *Creative visualisation: use of the power of your imagination to create what you want in your life.* Bantam, 1982

HEWITT, James *Meditation.* Hodder & Stoughton, 1978

ORNSTEIN, Robert E *The psychology of consciousness.* Cape, 1975

STEVENS, John O *Awareness.* Bantam, 1973

Chapter 8

COMFORT, Alex *The joy of sex: gourmet guide to lovemaking.* 2nd ed. Mitchell Beazley, 1983

MASTERS, William Howell and JOHNSON, Virginia Eshelman *Human sexual response.* Churchill, 1966

RAINER, Jerome and RAINER, Julia *Sexual adventure in marriage.* Panther, 1967

Chapter 9

BERNE, Eric *Games people play: psychology of human relationship.* Penguin, 1970

HARRIS, Thomas A *I'm Ok, you're OK.* Pan, 1973

LAING, Ronald *Knots*. New ed. Penguin, 1972
MILLER, Sherod and others *Couple workbook*. Interpersonal
Communication Program Publications, 1976
SKYNNER, Robin and CLEESE, John *Families and how to survive
them*. New ed. Methuen, 1984
WILSON, Colin *The outsider*. Gollancz, 1956 (Pan, 1978, paper)

Chapter 10
HODGKINSON, Liz *The working woman's guide*. Thorsons, 1985
MELHUISH, Andrew *Work and health* New ed. Penguin, 1982

Chapter 11
BRITISH MEDICAL ASSOCIATION *The medical effects of nuclear
war: report*. Wiley, 1983
CARSON, Rachel *Silent spring*. New ed. Pelican, 1982
EHRLICH, Paul Ralph *Population bomb*. Pan, 1971
McKOORMICK, John *The user's guide to the environment*. Kogan
Page, 1985
MEADOWS, Donella H and others. *Limits to growth: a report for
the Club of Rome's project to the predicament of mankind*. Signet,
1972
ROBERTSON, James *The sane alternative: a choice of futures*. 2nd
ed. The author, 1983
WARD, Barbara and DUBOS, Rene *Only one earth*. Penguin,
1972

Chapter 12
BERGER, John and ROWLANCE, Christopher, eds. *About time*.
Cape, 1985
CUPITT, Don *The sea of faith: Christianity in charge*. BBC, 1985
DOSSEY, L *Space, time and medicine*. Routledge & Kegan Paul,
1982
FRENCH, Reginald Michael *The Way of the Pilgrim*. Bantam
1974
HAPPOLD, F C *Mysticism*. Revised ed. Penguin, 1965
KUBLER-ROSS, Elisabeth *Living with death and dying*. Souvenir
Press, 1982
ORNSTEIN, Robert E *On the experience of time*. Penguin, 1969
SALMON, Phillida *Living in time: new look at personal
development*. Dent, 1985
VAN FRANZ, Marie Louise *Time: patterns of flow and return*.
Thames & Hudson, 1979

Index